Professional Responsibility in Dentistry

Professional Responsibility in Dentistry

A Practical Guide to Law and Ethics

Joseph P. Graskemper, DDS, JD

Second Edition

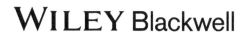

Library of Congress Cataloging-in-Publication Data
Names: Graskemper, Joseph P., author.
Title: Professional responsibility in dentistry : a practical guide to law
    and ethics / Joseph P. Graskemper, DDS, JD.
Description: Second edition. | Hoboken, NJ : John Wiley & Sons, 2023. |
    Includes bibliographical references and index.
Identifiers: LCCN 2022049699 (print) | LCCN 2022049700 (ebook) | ISBN
    9781119830061 (paperback) | ISBN 9781119830078 (pdf) | ISBN
    9781119830085 (epub)
Subjects: LCSH: Dental laws and legislation—United States. | Dental
    ethics—United States.
Classification: LCC KF2910.D32 G73 2023 (print) | LCC KF2910.D32 (ebook) |
    DDC 344.7304/13—dc23/eng/20221019
LC record available at https://lccn.loc.gov/2022049699
LC ebook record available at https://lccn.loc.gov/2022049700

Cover Images: © Drazen Zigic/Getty Images, © SolisImages/Getty Images
Cover Design by Wiley

Set in 9.5/12.5pt STIXTwoText by Integra Software Services Pvt. Ltd, Pondicherry, India
Printed and bound by CPI Group (UK) Ltd, Croydon, CR0 4YY

C118345_260123

Contents

Preface

This book is a result of a need to bring together the "soft subjects" of dental law, dental ethics, professionalism, risk management, and practice management. Dentists, being science-oriented, tend to enjoy concise, fact-based information as found in many science courses. The "soft subjects" do not always lend themselves to simple, black and white, concise answers requiring as little discussion as is involved with the fit of a crown. Dentists, having a definitive and result-oriented training, rely on factual results. The "soft subjects" do not lend themselves to a discussion ending with exact results

This book presents a fact-based presentation in a guidebook format that science-oriented dentists are used to. The "true cases" are from over 40 years of practice on both East and West Coasts, legal and practice management consultations, and expert witnessing experiences. The true cases make the "soft subjects" of dentistry, which are often boring and of little interest to dentists, more practical and interesting. It is a little touch of reality by which the material presented may be applied to discussion and make an impact on the practicality of the "soft subjects" to the actual practice of dentistry.

These subjects are normally taught individually and in a vacuum, while they are in reality very much integrated into each other. When I was asked to take over the Dental Law class and combine it with the Dental Ethics and Professionalism class it became a challenge. While developing the combined courses, many crossover issues became more apparent than I had originally anticipated. The course material also started to intersect with practice management issues. I then renamed the courses to be Professional Responsibility I and II to better identify the actual subject matter discussed: Dental Law, Ethics, Professionalism, Risk Management, and Practice Management. Normally these subjects are taught separately, but must be utilized together in dental practice. The dental student, given the different pieces of professional responsibility separately in a vacuum, is then left to put the pieces together after graduation. This book brings the various "soft subject" concepts, ideas, rules, and regulations together in a practical guidebook format.

With the application of issues, rules, analysis, and conclusion (IRAC) to the many dental legal, ethical, professional, risk management, and practice management issues confronting a dentist as practitioner, employer/employee, educator, and/or business owner, or to any of the true cases, a discussion may be had regarding the intermingling of these "soft subjects" as they relate to the actual practice of dentistry and not as separate entities with their separate concepts and patterns of thought.

In this second edition, many new issues have come forth from social media to employee management. Attention has been given to update the entire book to make it as useful as possible to the new dentist as well as the seasoned professional.

It should be pointed out that many of the rules, regulations, and laws may be different in the jurisdiction in which you practice; as such, you should always retain proper legal, tax, or practice management advice.

Joseph Graskemper, DDS, JD

Acknowledgments

I again dedicate this second edition to Tara, the love of my life, my ever-caring wife. Thank you for being my companion while I pursued my dreams of obtaining a law degree and for working side-by-side with me developing our successful multispecialty dental practice – all while raising a family and then relocating across the country from California to New York. I highly value and appreciate your outstanding encouragement and support during the writing of this book. Throughout my "not listening", "I'll be right there" conversations and the most recent famous "going to the basement for a little while to write" (usually for a couple of hours), you always were understanding.

I would also like to admire our children and their spouses Joe and Allie, Gena, and Paige and Doug, who have given me much needed encouragement, patience, and understanding while they, themselves, have continued down their individual roads to success.

And to my office staff, Michele Yalamas, RDH, Erin Condit RDH, Cathy Perten, and Sandra Richiusa, for constantly hearing "I'll be there in a minute" while I continued to type and they explained to the waiting patient I'll just be a moment longer.

I would also like to acknowledge those whom I may not have identified sooner and from whom I have drawn my conclusions and opinions, and apologize in advance of any inadvertent omission.

About the Author

Joseph P. Graskemper (DDS, JD, DABLM, FAGD, FAES, FICOI, FASO, FCLM, FACD) currently practices full-time in Bellport, New York, and is an associate clinical professor at Stony Brook School of Dental Medicine, teaching professionalism, ethics, and risk management. His previous practice experience includes being the sole owner of a fee-for-service multi-specialty group practice in La Jolla, California, where he was also the owner of a full-service dental lab and an advertising agency for dentists. He was the Past Director of Professional Responsibility courses. Dr. Graskemper has been awarded six fellowships by the following organizations – Academy of General Dentistry, American Endodontic Society, International Congress of Oral Implantologists, American Society of Osseointegration, American College of Legal Medicine, and American College of Dentists. He is also a diplomat in the American Board of Legal Medicine, past board member of the International Dental Ethics and Law Society, American College of Legal Medicine (past President-Elect), and the Suffolk County Dental Society. He also provides practice management consulting, expert witness testimony, and has served as a consultant to State Dental Boards. Dr. Graskemper has authored many peer-reviewed articles, lectured and published nationally and internationally, and authored the companion book: "Leadership and Communication in Dentistry." He may be reached at drjosephddsjd@gmail.com for comments, consultations, or as a speaker.

Part I

Legal Concepts

1

The Lawsuit

A lawsuit starts when you receive a complaint letter from the patient or the attorney that states that you are being sued. But before discussing this we must examine why patients sue. I have found that there are basically two reasons: (1) the patient has allegedly been harmed in some manner as a result of your treatment or nontreatment, and (2) the patient wants money. The problem the patient may have, may not even pertain to dentistry, as seen in True Case 1.

True Case 1: Miscarriage due to endodontics

A healthy, pregnant woman in her 30s, in the beginning of her second trimester with no complications, came into the office with pain. She was referred to a board-certified endodontist who practiced part-time in the dental practice. A therapeutic pulpotomy was preformed. The patient was still having pain and went to another dentist, who reopened the tooth and performed a pulpectomy using endodontic files. The patient then had a miscarriage. The owner of the original dental office and the endodontist were sued for malpractice, causing the miscarriage (wrongful death) and emotional distress. The case was settled out of court at an arbitration hearing in favor of the defendant dentists. It was found that the subsequent treating dentist had separated a file resulting in loss of tooth.

The Complaint

The complaint letter will state many things that you have allegedly done to harm the patient. As seen from the case above, the patient and her attorney, who happened to be her uncle, blamed the dentists for the miscarriage. An attorney's letter will not only state your failure to follow a procedure's protocol and the standard of care but can also include complaints about a failure to refer, a failure to diagnose, or emotional distress. Remember, anyone can sue anybody at any time for anything for any amount. It does not mean the defendant did anything wrong or that the plaintiff will automatically win.

   Once the complaint letter has been received, what should you do? You should notify your malpractice carrier. However, before you notify them, be sure to recognize the difference between an incident and a claim. An "incident" is often called a "near miss" – for example, two airplanes passing each other closely. A "claim" is a hit – a collision. If the letter is from a disgruntled patient,

Professional Responsibility in Dentistry: A Practical Guide to Law and Ethics, Second Edition. Joseph P. Graskemper.
© 2023 John Wiley & Sons, Inc. Published 2023 by John Wiley & Sons, Inc.

try to decide if it is a manageable situation (see Chapter 14). If not, you should contact your insurance company. The insurance company would prefer that you always contact them so they may assist you and keep track of your troubled patient relations. Every time you contact your insurance company it is placed in your record. If you contact them too many times, it indicates to the insurance company that you have problems within the office with patient communications, patient finances, and/or procedure protocols. Depending on the number and severity of your "incidents," the insurance company may either increase your premium or drop you because you have troubled patient relations or questionable treatment outcomes. If the letter is from an attorney's office, you must call your insurance company.

Once you receive the complaint letter, retrieve the record from the main office filing system. As soon as possible, write down in your own words what happened on a separate piece of paper and keep it separate from the patient file. This is your work product and is not part of the patient's treatment record. Do not change anything in the record as was done in True Case 2.

True Case 2: Changing the chart

Having been an expert witness many times, I must not fail to share the following experience. During the trial of a dentist in which I was the expert witness for the defendant dentist, the patient's attorney asked me if I would read what was on the top of page 3. The dentist's attorney had just gone through the record with me while I was on the witness stand to show how complete the patient's dental record was and how the dentist had followed the standard of care and all treatment protocols, thus the patient really did not have much of a case. The jury, I believe, was in full understanding that the dentist treated the patient properly. Now looking on the top of page 3, I read to the patient's attorney what I saw. He replied, "No, above that." There was nothing above that on my copy. He proceeded to show me and the jury his copy on which the dentist had made changes, after many copies had been made by both parties in preparation for the trial. He lost the case significantly due to altering the patient's record after some copies were already made.

Do not talk to anyone outside of your spouse and your staff. This will be a very emotional time that will lead to some self-doubt and second-guessing. Reassure yourself by reviewing your records to confirm you have followed all treatment protocols and the standard of care. Do not discuss the pending lawsuit with your colleagues or study club. Do not try to contact the patient or the patient's attorney.

After you contact the insurance company, they will assign you a claims administrator and an attorney, if needed. The sooner you contact the insurance company regarding a claim, the better the chance of success. The attorney assigned to you should be familiar with dental terminology and dental malpractice lawsuits. This attorney is usually on retainer with the insurance company. If the case is beyond the limits of your policy, be sure to also have your own personal attorney. Most times this is not necessary.

True Case 3: Saving the case for trial

At an arbitration hearing, which may occur before a trial, where I was the expert witness for the dentist, a question of comparative negligence (to be covered later – the patient is partly responsible for the damages) was not asked. While walking back to the dentist's attorney's office, I asked him why he did not ask several questions that would have easily, in my opinion, settled the case in the dentist's favor. His reply was that he was going to save those questions for the trial!

Hence it is important for dentists to have a basic understanding of the legalities that apply to the practice of dentistry.

Some states have a claims committee within their state dental association [1]. These claims committees may be asked by the insurance company to review the evidence of the case and to render an opinion as to whether to settle or to defend a case. This type of review may be available only to dental association members. You may still decide to defend the case even if the committee recommends settlement. That decision depends on you, your case, and the type of malpractice insurance you have (to be discussed in Chapter 20).

Examination before Trial

The next thing to happen is the examination before trial (EBT), also described as the discovery phase. The EBT may include interrogatories and depositions. Arbitration and settlement hearings may also occur prior to an actual trial. Interrogatories are long, written questionnaires about you and the dental care you provided for the plaintiff/patient. This is then followed by depositions. These are fact-finding, direct questionings of each party to the lawsuit by the opposing attorney. These are taken under oath and with a court reporter. Both attorneys are usually present, but only one party, the dentist/defendant or the patient/plaintiff, is deposed at a time. You will be given a copy of the deposition and asked to make any corrections and sign it. Be sure to check it closely for errors because they do occur, and once it is signed you cannot change it. Those errors, if of significant importance, may be held against you if you go to trial. Both parties, depending on the jurisdiction, may then agree to an arbitration. There are binding and nonbinding arbitrations. A binding arbitration is where both parties agree that the result will be the end of the lawsuit. The nonbinding arbitration still leaves the avenue open to further litigate the case if either party feels the result of the arbitration was not fair. Both types of arbitration are usually held with both parties and their attorneys, with a retired judge or highly experienced attorney who is familiar with malpractice acting as the arbitrator. Settlement conferences are sometimes held when the amount of damages has not been agreed upon but both parties have resolved the liability question of the case. At these various fact-finding discovery proceedings, the attorneys will try to

1) Find out the facts that you know and explain your patient records.
2) Evaluate your credibility and whether you would make a good, impressionable witness.
3) Use leading questions to catch you at some discrepancy between your interrogatory and deposition (see Chapter 14).

Almost all dental malpractice cases take place within the state court system. There are basically three levels of courts within each state: trial court, appellate court, and state supreme court. Most dental malpractice cases are resolved at the trial court level, but sometimes they make it to the court of appeals. It should be noted that many dental lawsuits are settled before an actual trial starts due to the time and cost of a trial. At the trial level, there is usually a judge and jury, with some jurisdictions allowing a jury by request.

Please keep in mind that judges and juries are humans who have biases and ideas of justice and fairness with which you may not agree. No matter how solid a case may seem, no one can predict how a trial will be resolved. In addition to the talents of each attorney and the credibility of the dentist and the patient/plaintiff, the expert witness for each side also affects the outcome of a trial. If the attorney does not ask the right questions for the expert to properly answer, the most solid of cases may be lost.

You should also be aware of the small claims court in your jurisdiction. The limits on damages are much lower but have often been used by the patient to get a refund of money or by the dentist to collect past due balances for treatment rendered. This will be discussed more under patient finances (see Chapter 21).

The Results

The results of the lawsuit have varying consequences. If you win your case or is settled out of court, there is still an impact on you and your practice. Financially, you have lost time out of the office resulting in lost production. Your malpractice insurance premium may increase or even possibly be dropped by your insurer. The plaintiff/patient may appeal the case.

If you lose your case, you still lost production. If you signed a waiver to settle with your malpractice insurer, decided to go to trial against the insurer's request to settle, you will most likely have to pay any amount over the insurance company's offer to settle to fulfil the court's decided amount of damages out of your own pocket. That amount over the insurer's settlement amount will not be covered by your insurance (see Chapter 20). There is also the risk of insurance premiums being increased or even dropped. Any money paid as a result of a claim must be reported to the National Practitioner Data Bank (NPDB).

There is also the emotional distress on you. There is even a syndrome called Medical Malpractice Stress Syndrome (MMSS) that brings attention to the impact on a health care provider when sued for malpractice. Litigation distress may directly contribute to physical illness, dissatisfaction with dental practice leading to burnout (see Chapter 12 – Leadership and Communication in Dentistry), and early retirement. The excessive worry that may last over six months, includes restlessness, tiredness, difficulty concentrating, irritability, insomnia, anger, loneliness, loss of self-esteem, and insecure in your ability and competency to make decisions in patient care [2]. If you are sued, you must continually reassure yourself that being sued for malpractice is a predictable hazard of clinical practice. You will become hesitant to continue to use the treatment strategy, technique, or material that is of issue in the lawsuit. You should re-evaluate and reassure yourself regarding your skills and talents.

In cases that are sizable, the Office of Professional Discipline (OPD) may review the case, investigate, and possibly place sanctions on the dentist's license.

A major dental malpractice insurer reports that the average cost of a malpractice lawsuit against a dental professional including legal defense is $137,497, which is a 30.5% increase in costs over a 5-year review (2016–2020). The claims against general dentists increased 30.5% and specialists

26.6%. General dentists accounted for 86.7% of claims. The procedure most cited for incurring liability is surgical extractions among all providers. However, allegations causing the highest claim costs are implants, due to the high costs of treatment, damages, and repair. The top five claims for dental procedures were found to be:

1) Implant surgery/placement
2) Root canal therapy
3) Surgical extractions
4) Crowns
5) Simple extraction

The increasing severity of claim costs can be attributed, in part, to social inflammation, which is the growth of liability/litigation risks and costs. This rate of growth is more rapid than what could be explained by general economic inflation, and there are a number of potential drivers of the rate of growth: sophisticated plaintiff attorney strategies, tort reform rollbacks, and the complexity of patient needs [3]. These influences will continue with the increase of high-cost procedures and the reduced trust in the doctor-patient relationship with corporate dental organizations seeking to become the primary dental care provider.

References

1 https://www.sddsny.org/about-us/leadership/committees, accessed November 13, 2022.

2 S. Sanbar and Marvin Firestone, *Legal Medicine and Medical Ethics*, 9th Edition, Chapter 5, p. 5, Law And Medicine Publication, 2015.

3 CNA, *Dental Professional Liability Claim Report*, 2nd Edition, Affinity Insurance Services, Fort Washington, 2021.

2

The Regulation of Dentistry

The regulation of dentistry is provided by federal as well as state laws. Federal laws and regulations are applied to all dentists. However, state laws, while many are identical to each other in some aspects, apply only in the state in which they have been enacted. So, throughout this discussion of the regulation of dentistry, be sure to always know the state version of the regulation in question. What may be legal in one state may be illegal in another state. For example, in Illinois, all removable appliances "shall be marked with the name or social security number, or both, of the patient for whom the prosthesis is intended. The markings shall be done during fabrication and shall be permanent, legible, and cosmetically acceptable" [1]. In California, "Every complete upper and lower denture fabricated by a licensed dentist, or pursuant to the dentist's work order, shall be marked with the patient's name or social security number, unless the patient objects" [2]. Then, in New York, it is stated a little differently: "Every dentist licensed in this state ... shall offer to the patient for whom the prosthesis is intended the opportunity to have such prosthesis marked with the patient's name or initials" [3]. As you can see, every state in regulating dentists has similar intentions of safeguarding the public, as seen here by attempting to prevent the loss of dental prostheses. However, each state will implement those safeguards in a slightly different manner

There are many facets to the regulation of dentistry: Statutes, Rules and Regulations, Civil, Institutional Rules, and Codes of Ethics. This chapter draws attention to the statutes, rules and regulations. Civil, which pertain to malpractice (Torts) and contracts, Institutional Rules and Codes of Ethics are found in following chapters.

Most states regulate the dental profession through a Dental Practice Act. The regulation of dentistry in most states usually falls under the purview of the State Board of Dentistry or the Board of Dental Examiners. The enforcement of the dental practice act is provided differently by each state. In Illinois, the Illinois State Dental Act is enforced by the Illinois Department of Professional Regulation [4]. In California, enforcement is through the Department of Consumer Affairs [5], while in New York, it is through the Office of Professional Discipline. New York actually has three agencies with administrative powers. The New York Board of Regents presides over the New York State Education Department, which oversees the preparation, licensure, and practice of the professions through the Office of the Professions, which then regulates dentistry through the State Board of Dentistry, which adopts neither rules nor regulations. It is charged instead with three responsibilities:

1) To serve as an examining body recommending licensure as dentists to the State Education Department.

Professional Responsibility in Dentistry: A Practical Guide to Law and Ethics, Second Edition. Joseph P. Graskemper.
© 2023 John Wiley & Sons, Inc. Published 2023 by John Wiley & Sons, Inc.

2) To advise the state legislature, the Commissioner of Education, and the Board of Regents on dental matters, e.g., proposed changes and additions to the dental practice act.
3) To serve as an administrative body to hear violations of rules and regulations through the Office of Professional Discipline and to report its findings to the Board of Regents [6].

These agencies have a far-reaching capacity in the investigation of a dentist. In most jurisdictions, any conviction, misdemeanor or felony (DUI, failure to file taxes, insurance billing fraud) may go to the agency for review.

These investigative agencies usually have the power to recommend suspension, to limit scope of practice, and/or to revoke a dentist's license to the state board of dentistry. These agencies are very powerful in having the power to recommend revocation of one's license; in a lawsuit, only money damages are imposed on the dentist.

In the determination of a penalty the investigative agency will look at:

1) The alleged harm/damages to the patient.
2) The dentist having any prior history of misconduct.
3) The duration and extent of the misconduct.
4) The proximity or connectiveness of the misconduct to the harm.
5) The impact of the penalty on the dentist.
6) The mitigating and aggregating factors.

Most jurisdictions provide a reporting procedure that allows the regulatory agencies to review court proceedings. In the review of such proceedings, the agency may decide further investigation and possibly restrictive action is needed to protect the public from the offending dentist. The agency may also receive complaints directly from a patient, employee, or the general public anonymously regarding a dentist. In the interest of protecting the public, most jurisdictions provide statutes that allow and sometimes demand these agencies to investigate such a complaint, even if it is anonymous. Such agencies, although they are required to investigate, do not have the right to go on a "fishing expedition" through your office. Hence, if you receive a letter from your state agency, take it very seriously.

True Case 4: Dental state board case of fractured porcelain

A dentist received a letter from the state's investigative agency. In this case it was the New York State Office of Professional Discipline. It had received a complaint directly from a patient. In the complaint, the patient stated that a crown was placed approximately two years prior to the problem he encountered. The porcelain fractured off his lower right molar crown (#30). A letter was sent to the dentist informing him that a complaint was made to the agency and that the agency was investigating the complaint. They requested from the dentist a statement and copies of all the patient's records. All requested information was supplied with the help of an attorney knowledgeable in such proceedings. It was pointed out that the dentist was never informed by the patient that there was a problem, that the patient could have had trauma from biting or chewing abnormally hard food or an object, and that it is the dentist's habit and custom to help such patients by remaking the crown at no charge if needed, within a reasonable time period. The agency found in favor of the dentist.

As seen in True Case 4, you can never predict when the investigative agency in your jurisdiction may be contacting you. If this does happen, *you do have rights*. You have the right to protect your interests. You have the right to legal counsel. You have the right to schedule an office visit and not be forced to allow immediate access to your office and records. In other words, if they are knocking at your door, you do not have to let them in; you may refuse access on the basis they are interfering with your current patient care. You may ask them to schedule an office visit. (Caveat: Only if public safety is not in question.) Be sure to seek an attorney who is very familiar with the agency's procedure to properly advise and protect you. Most state dental associations or dental malpractice insurance companies have contacts available for such a situation. Depending on the state, most dental malpractice insurance policies contain provisions for covering the legal costs up to a certain limit.

The unintended consequences of a settlement, after OPD is done reviewing and finalizing the action against the dentist, the case may be sent to the Medicaid Inspector General, whether or not the dentist is a Medicaid provider. If it is sent, then it may be decided that the dentist has a Disqualified Status, whereby affecting the dentist's participation as a Medicaid provider or faculty status, because most schools accept Medicaid. Any action by OPD will be on your record forever.

Federal Oversight

The various, approximately 53 (including Puerto Rico, the Virgin Islands, and the District of Columbia), state dental practice acts and their accompanying rules, regulations, and statutes govern and provide oversight of licensure, continuing education, permits, auxiliary dental personnel, exemptions, special provisions, advertising, referrals, professional misconduct, and unprofessional conduct, along with other areas of dental care. Before exploring these rules and regulations, we should first look at the federal oversight of providing dental health care. There are many nondental federal agencies that affect the way you practice dentistry: Occupational Safety and Health Administration (OSHA), Center for Disease Control (CDC), Food and Drug Administration (FDA), Social Security Administration/Medicaid, and the Environmental Protection Agency (EPA) to name just a few. There are also the Americans with Disabilities Act and the National Practitioners Data Bank (NPDB).

OSHA

The Occupational Safety and Health Administration was established to protect the employee in the workplace. This became especially apparent and applicable to dentistry in the 1980s when new regulations were developed in response to the discovery and rapid spread of the HIV and AIDS. Because some health care providers refused to treat HIV/AIDS positive patients due to fear of contracting the disease, OSHA issued regulations and standards to protect all health care workers, including those in a dental setting. The CDC, in 1991 and working with OSHA, set guidelines for all health care workers to prevent further spread of diseases and injuries. All employees, part-time included, must be offered, at no cost to the employee, vaccination for hepatitis within 10 days of employment. It also provided what are now known as "universal precautions" for all health care workers to prevent the transmission of infectious diseases [7].

Therefore, dentists must properly wash hands before and after patient treatment, during which they must wear gloves, mask, protective eyewear, and fluid-resistant gown. Some dentists, along with other health care workers, at that time still held the position that their offices were private and should be allowed to treat only those whom they wish. In other words, they wanted to continue to discriminate against HIV/AIDS-positive patients in their practices. The passing of the Americans with Disabilities Act firmly stated that the private offices of health care providers (dentists included) were "places of public accommodation" and therefore must adhere to the federal antidiscrimination laws [7]. It also required all health care providers to treat all patients in the same manner, regardless of color, creed, religion, national origin, or disability, with special confidentiality of patients with HIV/AIDS. It made very clear that the construction of health care facilities must meet requirements for the handicapped. There were also special hiring regulations put in place if there are 15 or more employees. The act also governed employees. Employees cannot refuse to treat patients with HIV/AIDS; and if they do so, the employer may fire those employees who refuse to treat due to violation of this act. Employees with HIV/AIDS cannot be fired and should be reassigned and given a position without direct patient care. It should be pointed out that the CDC only gives guidelines, which are recommendations and not requirements. It has no enforcement powers. However, OSHA does have enforcement powers and exercises those powers by converting CDC guidelines into enforceable regulations. Those regulations were incorporated into the Postal Workers and Transportation Appropriations Act and made law. It imposes a penalty of loss or suspension of professional license if a health care professional is not compliant with the guidelines of the CDC. It should be pointed out that failure to comply would not just result in a penalty or fine but actual possible loss of your license.

There are many OSHA/Infection Control Manuals available on the market to help set up protocol in the dental office. It should include, but not limited to:

1) Written documentation of office policies.
2) Exposure control precautions, sharps disposal policy.
3) Hepatitis vaccination employee documentation.
4) Housekeeping/infection control protocol for the entire office.
5) Blood-borne pathogens standards and training.
6) OSHA employee information poster.
7) Post-exposure protocol.
8) Maintain material safety data sheets (MSDS).
9) Office records, which should include an office injury report (everything from paper cuts to needle-sticks).

With the Covid 19 epidemic erupting in 2019, many changing regulations affecting dental offices were put in place by CDC and OSHA; such as safe distancing, proper protection (N95, KN95, Level 3) level mask wearing, and even required vaccination with rarely any exceptions allowed. Many dental offices placed environmental air hygiene equipment (air scrubbers, Hepa filters, Hepa air recirculators to name a few) in their office to help keep patients safe.

Employee injury and illness records must be kept for 30 years, all others for 3 years. The OSHA (including the Material Safety Data Sheets, MSDS)/Infection Control/Blood-borne Pathogens manual must be made easily available to the employees without their having to ask. Record keeping, as seen in True Case 5, must be kept up in a timely and complete manner (see Chapter 9).

True Case 5: OSHA

In the early 1980s, when this agency was developing dental office oversight, OSHA offered to come into your office to check on your compliance. Anything that was found to be noncompliant would not result in a fine as long as the dentist rectified the problem in a timely manner. A dentist (me) thought it was a good idea. Having made sure all nine operatories and the central sterilization area were prepared for the review, I invited OSHA into my practice. When the OSHA agents came, they spent about 20 minutes walking through the operatories and about 6 hours going through my files in the business office. Their biggest finding, which was unexpected, was that our Injury Report Log was not posted in the office and was not filled out. They could not believe that even a paper cut hadn't happened in the office. They were more concerned about proper reports, recorded meetings and training sessions, and identification of materials (MSDS).

FDA/DEA/EPA

The FDA and the Drug Enforcement Administration (DEA), which is under the jurisdiction of the Department of Justice, govern the medications and drugs for which you write prescriptions. To write prescriptions, you will need to apply for a DEA number, which will allow you to write class 2, 3, 4, and 5 drug prescriptions. Many states have put in place an e-script regulation that all prescriptions must be electronically sent to the pharmacy with many safeguards for prescribing narcotics. The Environmental Protection Agency (EPA) also regulates dentistry because of the hazardous wastes generated in dentistry. The regulation requires most general dentists to install an amalgam separator to prevent the mercury contained in dental amalgam from entering the air, water, and land. Dental offices that place or remove amalgam must operate and maintain an amalgam separator and must not discharge scrap amalgam or use certain kinds of line cleaners [8]. It requires an amalgam separator with a filter that must be replaced by an authorized company on a timely basis as required by the state law. These disposal rules and regulations are dependent on your respective state laws. The New York State Dental Mercury and Amalgam Recycling Law states that "no dentist shall use or possess elemental mercury in the practice unless such elemental mercury is contained in appropriate pre-encapsulated capsules specifically designed for the mixing of dental amalgam. All dentists shall recycle any elemental mercury, and dental amalgam waste generated in their dental practices in accordance with rules and regulations established by the commissioner" [9]. Hazardous wastes, which also include medical/biological waste, may also include but are not limited to: used and unused amalgam fragments, radiographic solutions, various sharps (needles, endodontic files, scalpels, etc.), blood-soaked gauze, and/or cotton, body parts (extracted teeth, gingival tissue, bone, etc.), and expired dental medicaments. Each of these items may require separate disposal by an authorized/certified transporter and disposal company. The EPA also oversees the efficacy of the chemicals used to disinfect the office. Be sure you are using properly identified chemicals, per OSHA regulations, in your infection control protocol.

There are many other agencies within each state that also regulate dentistry, such as the New York State Department of Health-regulated inspection of radiation equipment under the Bureau of Environmental Radiation Protection. In California, radiation equipment must comply with the California Radiation Control Regulations (Title 17, Cal. Code Regs., commencing with section

30100) and it is overseen by the Department of Health Services [10]. Due to each state having its own authority to regulate radiation equipment and other state-interested areas in health care, such as labor/employment laws, nondentist ownership of a dental practice, and independent contractor/employee associateship, it is beyond the scope of this book to discuss the differences of each state's various regulations.

NPDB

The National Practitioners Data Bank (NPDB) was originally formed in 1990 to collect information regarding impaired or incompetent physicians and dentists and those who engaged in unprofessional behavior [11]. Information is collected from insurance companies, which must report settlements within 30 days of payment of a malpractice suit. Hospitals and licensing agencies, such as state dental boards, must report any actions that affect a dentist's ability to perform, such as a limited, suspended, or revoked license. Courts also must report court-ordered malpractice judgments to the NPDB. Additionally, individual dentists must report any payment of money to a patient per the patient's written request. Any exchange of money resulting from a written request or claim based on health care services is reportable, such as a malpractice insurer settlement payment. To be reportable, there must be an exchange of money that was paid by an entity (not personal) for the benefit of health care practitioner due to a written claim or demand for money that is based on a failure to provide service properly. All these elements must be satisfied for the case to be reportable. This information is then made available to hospitals, health care facilities, and licensing agencies such as dental state boards. It is not available to insurance companies, attorneys, or patients. You should receive a Practitioner Notification Document every time a report has been filed with the NPDB regarding yourself [12]. However, due to the public's demand for more information and easy Internet access to information, this may change. Therefore, if the situation arises in which you must refund money to a patient, be sure of three major aspects:

1) Do it before the patient asks for it in writing.
2) Payment is made personally and not through an insurance company or corporation if possible.
3) You must get a signed Release of Claims with an antidefamation clause (that meets your state's criteria) before release of any money or writing a check.
4) Check with your local attorney and your malpractice insurance company as to whether a refund may be used against you in a court of law, even with a signed release of claims.

It is not reportable if you give a waiver of the fees, redoing the work, or the patient does not ask for money.

HIPAA

The Health Insurance Portability and Accountability Act (HIPAA) was passed in 1996 by Congress to:

1) Protect and enhance the rights of consumers to access their health information.

2) Improve the quality of health care by restoring trust in the health care system by mandating a fraud and abuse control program.
3) Improve the efficiency and effectiveness of health care delivery.

HIPAA's main purpose is to protect the confidentiality and privacy of the patient's health care information. In a typical 3–5-day hospital stay, an estimated 150 people have legitimate access to the patient's records. Under HIPPA, patients have the right to access, copy, inspect, and amend their health care information, to obtain an accounting of the right to request restrictions on disclosures, and to file complaints regarding their health care information. There are four rules under HIPAA:

1) The Privacy Rule for all patient information.
2) The Security Rule for safe-guarding electronic patient.
3) The Breach Notification Rule for notification to patients and government agencies that a breach has occurred.
4) The Enforcement Rule for oversight and investigations of HIPAA violations.

Under the Privacy Rule, you must inform the patient of your health care information privacy policy and have them sign the form. You must keep all patient information private and confidential.

1) You must have a health information privacy policy and procedures.
2) Patients must sign a "consent for use" and a "disclosure of health information" form.
3) Patients must sign an "acknowledgment of receipt of notice of privacy practices" form.

On the form there is also a place for the patient to sign a waiver of such forms. Without the patient's signature on these forms, you are not able to send any e-mails or recall/maintenance visit postcards. Any postal communication with the patient must then be done through a sealed envelope rather than a postcard. There is also the business associate agreement for any organization or person whom you engage to perform or assist you in which that assistance involves the use or disclosure of protected health care information created for or received from your office. These forms and compliance guides are easily available from numerous dental associations and societies.

Under the Security Rule, you must assess the risk and place safeguards to protect patient's electronic information, secure confidentiality and provide proper employee training. The Office of Civil Rights enforces HIPAA Security Rules. Texting is permissible but beware of the threat of not being secured. The text message must comply with the technical safe guards of the HIPAA Security Rule's "minimum necessary standards and the content of the message does not include any of the 18 Personal Identifiers":

1) Name.
2) Address (all geographic subdivisions smaller than state, including street address, city, county, and zip code).
3) All elements (except years) of dates related to an individual (including birthdate, admission date, discharge date, date of death, and exact age if over 89).
4) Telephone numbers.
5) Fax number.
6) Email address.
7) Social Security Number.
8) Medical record number.

9) Health plan beneficiary number.
10) Account number.
11) Certificate or license number.
12) Vehicle identifiers and serial numbers, including license plate numbers.
13) Device identifiers and serial numbers.
14) Web URL.
15) Internet Protocol (IP) Address.
16) Finger or voice print.
17) Photographic image – Photographic images are not limited to images of the face.
18) Any other characteristic that could uniquely identify the individual [13].

Ransomware is a type of malicious software (malware) that is designed to block access to a computer or a network of computers until a sum of money is paid for its release, as seen in True Case 6. There is no guarantee that the attackers will return the information access after payment is made. The attackers may mine your patient information while being held ransom even though payment was made.

True Case 6: Ransomware

Ransomware has become a true problem in security of patient information. In this case the dentist did not have a back up to the cloud or to a hard drive that is taken off-site. A demand was made for $10,000 for release of the office's computers. The dentist had to notify all patients that a breach had occurred. If he would have had a viable secure system that was properly backed up daily in a safe off-site location, he could have escaped the payment of $10,000.

The Breach Notification Rule requires you to notify the patients involved in the breach, as well as the federal government (US Department of Health and Human Services – HHS). If the breach affects more than 500 individuals, the media must also become involved in the notification process. Many states have breach notification laws that also must be followed. There is now insurance, which is highly advised, available to cover the expenses of the breach. It is very important to seek legal advice as soon as possible.

If a breach occurs there are six basic steps that must be followed.

1) Contain the breach – change all passwords, reroute to new network, restore with uninfected backup copy and abandon previous network.
2) Confirm the breach – find which computers affected, find origin of breach, identify all patients, employees, and vendors affected.
3) Obtain legal advice – must have knowledge of HIPAA violations.
4) Notification – Contact all affected by the breach including your malpractice carrier
5) Patient and Public Relations – Send a letter to all patients ASAP informing them of the breach and what is being done including if you are offering a free or discounted credit monitoring service.
6) Reset data security – upgrade firewalls, passwords, and backup systems.

Under the Enforcement Rule penalties can be severe. The penalties for noncompliance are based on the level of negligence and can range from $100 to $50,000 per violation (or per record), with a maximum penalty of $1.5 million per year for violations of an identical provision. Violations can also carry criminal charges that can result in jail time. The fines and charges are broken down into four tiers:

1) No knowledge – reasonably diligent
2) Reasonable cause – should have known
3) Unwilful neglect – corrected in 30 days
4) Willful neglect – not corrected in 30 days [14]

HIPAA also requires you to retain patient records for six years from the patient's last appointment or two years from the patient's death. There are also state laws that address the retention of patient records.

You must be careful when using electronic media to talk to patients. It must be secure and encrypted. Texting is considered a strict liability breach. All patient information and treatments are confidential. To encourage health care providers to adopt electronic health records and improved privacy and security protections for health care data, the HITECH Act enacted to give financial incentives to the health care providers.

In 2009, the Office of Civil Rights took over as the enforcer of the HIPAA Security Rules. Some of the violations that have been found are as follows:

Inadequate passwords.
Computers that did not log off users after inactivity.
Unencrypted laptops.
Outdated anti-virus software.
Unchanged default user identification and passwords.

TCPA

The Telephone Consumer Protection Act (TCPA) was an attempt to address the problem of unwanted telemarketing communications (especially third parties). It allows individuals to sue up to $1,500 for every phone call or text that violated the law. There is also the Telephone Sales Rule (TSR) that applies to phone calls and texts with a marketing or advertising message for a service. This can be applied to appointment reminders that also solicit or promote a dental service or treatment when the reminder is sent out. The patient must also agree to receive the electronic appointment reminder. Dentists must keep updated patient information regarding the want to receive the electronic reminder and the correct phone number or email address is current. Calling the wrong number frequently, as described in True Case 7, is a violation [15]. There are many companies offering the management of your recall, appointment reminders, and happy birthday greetings. Make sure they are keeping all information confidential, patient information and the patient's choice as to whether they wish to have electronic notifications correct. Even though they are a third party hired to make such notifications you as the owner of the practice will be held liable for mistakes.

True Case 7: Unsolicited texts

Ms. Hill v TLC Dental-Hollywood (S.D. Fla.) January 2020
   Ms. Hill claimed numerous unsolicited texts received on her cellphone were sent without her consent. The text stated "We are open today." Her damages included the depletion of the phone's battery, rendering the phone unusable, and diminished the phone's memory. The Federal Trade Commission (FTC) identified this as "real harm."

Licensure

Licensure is delegated to the individual states by which each state has the authority to regulate dentistry within its own jurisdiction. Most states are very similar in their requirements for licensure. All require passing the National Dental Board Examinations (Parts I and II). Most states require passing a state-specific clinical examination or regional board examination. This is currently a changing area in that there has been a consolidation of the clinical testing over the past years. At one time, some states would only accept their respective state clinical test. Almost all states are part of a regional clinical examination. New York, Delaware, and possibly others to follow, have even relieved the burden of a clinical examination and added the requirement of a one-year residency program (PGY1) that has a formal outcome assessment prior to licensure [16]. More states may opt to go with a residency requirement in lieu of a clinical examination in the future to relieve the burden of basing licensure on a few procedures viewed over a 1 to 2-day period. California recently passed AB 1524 to allow licensure via a dental school-based portfolio covering seven subject areas during their final year of dental school [17]. Some states also require a state-specific topic test normally dealing with the state's ethics and jurisprudence, rules, and regulations. Other requirements for licensure may include but are not limited to fingerprinting, age minimum, citizenship status, cardiopulmonary resuscitation (CPR) license, and fees.

Many, if not most, jurisdictions provide for licensure through reciprocity and/or licensure by credentials. Reciprocity is an agreement between two jurisdictions to honor the other's licensure. True reciprocity without any conditions is very rare. Most have some conditions that must be met to accept the other jurisdiction's licensure. Most jurisdictions favor licensure by credentials. There are usually criteria to be met that include, but may not be limited to, requirements of another jurisdiction, licensed in other jurisdiction a certain number of years (normally 3–5 years) and is in good standing, has not been subject to disciplinary action by any state in which he or she has been licensed, a signed release allowing disclosure of information from the NPDB, and has maintained and is able to document a certain number of hours of continuing education [18, 19].

There are limited permits that most jurisdictions allow for residencies and dental school faculty. These limited permits are usually renewable on a yearly basis and do not allow the limited permit holder to have a private practice. Some states, such as California, have different requirements for foreign-trained dentists [20].

Due to the mandated closure of many dental offices during the COVID-19 Pandemic, teledentistry became well used. However, if treating a patient out of state or referring to a dentist (radiologist or pathologist) via teledentistry, and that referred to dentist does not have a license in your state, you may be held liable for any mis-diagnoses/damages/malpractice by that dentist. Most states require a state license to practice dentistry in their state. There were some exceptions during the pandemic that remain for outlying underserved areas per the various state jurisdictions.

Continuing Education

In every dental practice act, there is a section detailing the need for continuing education. Every state has certain requirements that are one-time courses, repeatable courses, and a certain number of course hours needed to maintain licensure. A one-time course may include Child Abuse, Tobacco and Oral Cancer, and Dental Law and Ethics, as seen in New York [21]. Repeatable courses may include infection control, CPR, and dental law, as seen in California [22]. Many jurisdictions limit the number of continuing education hours that can be provided by self-instructional, or otherwise recorded, such as webinars [23, 24]. The number of continuing education hours needed varies in the number of hours and the period of time between license renewals by each jurisdiction.

For a course to be acceptable for continuing education credit in some jurisdictions, such as New York, it must relate to the practice of dentistry and the sponsor must have at least one full-time employee who works at least 30 hours per week [21]. In California, the instructor should have education or experience within the last five years in the subject being taught [25].

Most jurisdictions require that the courses are relevant to the treatment and care of patients [23]. The clinical courses must directly pertain to patient treatment and nonclinical courses must relate to the skills necessary to provide services and are supportive of clinical services rendered. Courses dealing with money management, personal health, and estate planning are normally not acceptable for continuing education [23, 25].

I-Stop (Internet System for Tracking Over-Prescribing)

New York along with many states has instituted an electronic prescription surveillance of the medications prescribed. It was set up to deter the overprescribing of narcotics and made the written prescription obsolete. A failure to not cooperate or comply would be investigated by the state's disciplinary investigative agency such as the Office of Profession Discipline (OPD) in New York. All prescribed and/or dispensed Schedule 2, 3, 4 controlled substances must be queried in the Drug Registry through the Health Commerce System Prescription Monitoring Program. When queried with the patient's name and birthdate, a reference number is given that should be entered into the patient's chart to show you did so as regulated. This is in additional to the electronic prescribing for non-scheduled drugs. If technically impossible to access the registry and the patient is in need to prevent adverse patient consequences, you are granted 72 hours to log onto the system and enter the medication. There are also limitations on the amount of a narcotic you may prescribe. Some states like New York allow only a seven-day limit on opioid prescriptions for the initial dose.

All 50 states have some form of Prescription Monitoring Program (PMP) or Prescription Drug Monitoring Program (PDMP). Some states, such as Nevada, mandate and highly regulate the use of such program which requires a complete review of a patient's entire medical history prior to writing an opioid prescription. Nevada prescription writers must access the PMP once at least every six months to review the practitioner's prescribing information and verify their continued access to the PMP [26]. Other states may only recommend the use of the PMP/PDMP.

Permits

Most jurisdictions allow for special permits that pertain to certain situations where the dentist is not in private practice. These special permits are normally for faculty of a dental school. Most states have extended these special permits to dental residents. Dentists with special permits are usually not allowed to be in private practice under these types of permits. Some states such as California and Illinois provide specialty licenses for those who have complied with the requirements of a specialty. Only those dentists who have met such requirements are allowed to use "practice limited to ...," "specialist in ...," or similar phrases. Currently, some dentists have promoted non-American Dental Association (ADA) recognized specialty areas of dentistry such as cosmetic dentistry, temporomandibular joint, and implant dentistry as being a specialty. These will be discussed under "unprofessional conduct" in Chapter 17.

A separate dental anesthesia permit/certificate may be needed to sedate a patient, depending on the state and the level of the patient's sedation. A complete discussion of sedation is beyond the scope of this book. There are four general categories of sedation: minimal, moderate, deep, and general. Minimal sedation is a minimally depressed level, where the patient fully retains all physical abilities; whereas deep/general sedation is an induced state of depressed consciousness or complete unconsciousness. Many states may require a certificate for all levels of sedation. On the other hand, other states may require a certification for any sedation beyond conscious sedation. Conscious sedation is described differently by each state such that a permit may be required. Nitrous oxide, with or without oral medication, is not considered by some states to be conscious sedation, if the margin of safety is wide enough such that the unintended loss of consciousness is unlikely [27]. On the other hand, many states do not require a permit for the use of nitrous oxide, but may require a course certification showing proper training and that a scavenger system be used. Due to the wide variance in state regulation, be sure to seek proper advice from your state board and your malpractice insurance carrier to confirm proper insurance coverage.

Professional Misconduct and Unprofessional Conduct

In states like New York, "professional misconduct" and "unprofessional conduct" are separately mentioned in their statutes [28, 29]. Professional misconduct is acting as a professional wrongly within the performance as a dentist and unprofessional conduct is conduct unbecoming of a professional. Other states like Illinois and California simply state "unprofessional conduct" [30, 31]. All states have some provision within their dental practice acts that list those acts that are considered unprofessional conduct. Normally included, but not limited to, in these statutes, rules, or regulations are:

1) Fraud in obtaining a license.
2) Abandonment of a patient.
3) Wilfully making or filing false records.
4) Delegating professional responsibilities to unqualified persons.
5) Advertising professional superiority.
6) Guaranteeing services.
7) Failing to file a report mandated by law such as Child Abuse Reporting.
8) Allowing auxiliary personnel to perform duties not authorized by law.
9) Exercising undue influence on a patient for financial gain.
10) Harassing, abusing, or intimidating a patient.
11) Practicing beyond the scope of your licensure by law.
12) Committing act of gross immorality.
13) Fee-splitting or a sharing of fees for referrals and other state specific situations.
14) Practicing while impaired, intoxicated, addicted, or under the influence of drugs.
15) Convicted of a crime at the level of a felony.
16) Failing to use accepted infection control techniques.
17) Failure to maintain proper patient records or altering patient records with the intent to deceive [29–31].

This is a good sample of actions that are considered unprofessional conduct; you can see the list is long and varied. If a dentist is found guilty of unprofessional conduct, the enforcing agency will suspend or revoke his or her license, restrict or limit the scope of practice, require restitution of fees to the licentiate's patients or those who received services, place a probationary term of limited or no practice, and/or require the licentiate to submit to an examination followed by care, counselling, or treatment. Failure to comply with the directive from the enforcing agency tends to be grounds for the license to be revoked. In other words, you lose your license. Once that happens, it is hard to get another license in another state due to the NPDB.

True Case 8: Forfeit of license

A dentist in California had approximately 10 alleged malpractice cases pending. The California State Dental Board, once aware of this, began its investigation of the dentist and the cases. While the investigation was proceeding, the dentist applied to another state for licensure. Once he was granted a license in the other state, he forfeited his California license to the California State Dental Board, thus making any action against his California license meaningless. This occurred prior to 1990, when the NPDB was formed; this situation should now no longer occur.

True Case 9: Lost his license

In 1996, a dental practice was sold wherein the selling dentist arranged to accept payment of the balance over a five-year period to facilitate the sale. Once the selling dentist relocated to another state, the buying dentist stopped all payments. During the legal pursuit to gain payment, the selling dentist found out that the buying dentist lost (forfeited) his license in another state several years prior. When the state dental board was questioned about granting a license to a dentist with numerous licensure problems, they replied that the buying dentist checked the "No" box that asks if there were any problems or pending investigations regarding his former licensures.

From True Cases 8 and 9, you can see that even state boards may miss the mark of doing due diligence in their granting licensure. Even with the NPDB being fully up and running, the information that was easily found by the selling dentist and was overlooked by the granting state board.

Auxiliary Personnel

Supervision of dental auxiliaries is found in most dental practice acts to be separated into direct and general supervision. In New York, in what is called "direct supervision," and in Illinois, in what is called "supervision," the dentist must examine and diagnose the patient, and authorize the procedure and the treatment performed by the auxiliary prior to the patient's dismissal [32, 33]. The dentist must be in the office but not necessarily in the treatment room at all times.

The term "general supervision" is used when the dentist's physical presence is not required during the performance of those procedures that are based on the instruction given by the dentist [34]. New York State regulations also specify that the dentist must have means to be readily available and exercises that degree of supervision appropriate to the circumstances [32]. The phrase "readily available" means within a few minutes of being physically present. It is a good idea to follow the statute not only because it is the law but because it also agrees with proper risk management guidelines (see Chapter 14) and is ethically in the patient's best interest (see Chapter 17).

Therefore, when providing supervision of a dental auxiliary be sure to know the extent of training of your assistant and hygienist, and what they are allowed to do in your jurisdiction. True Case 10 is just one example in which a dentist has allowed a dental auxiliary to perform treatment beyond their skill, competence, or what is allowed by law.

True Case 10: Assistant extracted tooth

A dentist on a very busy day was confronted by an emergency in which a child patient, from a long-standing family of patients, needed a deciduous tooth removed. The dental assistant, who was a dentist licensed in another country, told the dentist that it was just a baby tooth that was loose and needed to come out. The dentist, who was really busy and could not immediately tend to the emergency, told the assistant to go ahead and remove the very loose baby tooth. The tooth was removed. Several days later, the child patient had swelling and infection in the area of the extraction. The parent took the child to another dentist, who took a radiograph and found a retained fractured root. A lawsuit resulted. The dental board found the dentist at fault, resulting in actions against the dentist's license.

Dental assistants are usually uncertified/unregistered or certified/registered in expanded functions. There are some states that have different levels of certification/registration, but there are normally assistants with training who are allowed to perform certain limited patient treatments and assistants without training who are only allowed to provide support to the dentist. To be certified/registered, the assistant must have completed state-authorized schooling and passed an examination for licensure. When hiring an assistant, it is advisable to always ask for a copy of his or her license to assure that he or she has been properly trained and licensed. Even though an assistant may be licensed, you, the employer–dentist, will be held responsible for his or her treatment. This is found in statutes and dental practice acts under fiduciary duty and respondeat superior principles in law (see Chapter 15).

To be certified or registered in expanded functions varies widely by state as to which procedures are allowed. In California, registered dental assistants in expanded functions (RDAEF) may, with proper licensure, do the following: place cord retraction of gingivae for impressions, take impressions for final cast restorations, etch teeth, apply sealants, dry canals and fit final endodontic points, remove excess cement subgingivally, polish crowns, fabricate, size, and temporarily cement temporary crowns, and place bases and liners on sound dentin [35]. They may even obtain a prophy license that allows them to polish teeth. This is a partial listing for California. Rather than making a "laundry list" of various allowed procedures, New York regulations state that a certified assistant may not diagnose or perform surgical, irreversible procedures that would alter the hard or soft tissue. They also state that the certified dental assistant cannot do that which is included in the duties and responsibilities that are limited to the scope of dentistry or dental hygiene [36]. Thus, the certified dental assistant cannot go so far as to do those procedures that are already limited to others. This truly puts the responsibility on the employer–dentist to properly supervise and know the competency of his or her assistants. It is normally found in all states that the higher the degree of involvement the dental assistant has with the patient, the more formal training and examinations are needed and the more directly the dentist must supervise the assistant.

Recently, in California, there has been a widening of the scope of duties for the dental assistant. California now allows registered dental assistants in extended function 2 (RDA-EF2) to place all types of restorations direct and indirect, alloy and composite, including endodontic points [37]. Other states are sure to follow.

Dental hygienists are normally trained and licensed by individual states rather than regional boards. Usually listed in each dental practice act are the procedures that are allowed for dental hygienists. They include, but not limited to, scaling and root planning, polishing, sealants, fluoride treatments, subgingival irrigation, and placement of intrasulcular antibiotics. Normally the biggest differences are the level of individual practice settings, the level of local anesthesia allowed, and the use of nitrous oxide. Each state may differ greatly in allowing these functions, which may be considered to be expanded and requiring further testing/licensure for it. For example, New York allows only infiltration anesthesia, while California allows infiltration and inferior alveolar blocks.

Advertising

Advertising was not allowed until 1979, when the Federal Trade Commission (FTC) began to interpret existing bans on advertising by professionals as unfairly restricting competition [38]. Because organized dentistry did not support the FTC's decision, they fought hard to side step it by not allowing dentists to join organized dentistry if they advertized as seen in True Case 11. Finally in May 1999, the US Supreme Court upheld that the FTC has jurisdiction over non-profit organizations and that price advertising is allowed if it is exact, accurate, and easily verifiable. Advertising that is not in the public interest may include:

1) False, misleading, deceptive ads.
2) Guarantees of service.
3) Claims of cost not substantiated with proof.
4) Claims of professional superiority.
5) Offers, bonuses, or inducements other than a discount of an established fee.
6) Compensation to media representatives for professional publicity.

Testimonials and portrayals have recently come under the purview of the FTC. The FTC Revised Endorsement and Testimonial Guides state that "an endorsement means any advertising message that consumers are likely to believe reflects the opinions, beliefs, finding, or experiences of a party other than the sponsoring advertiser" [39]. The endorser must be a "bona fide user of [the product] at the time the endorsement was given" and the advertiser has good reason that the endorser continues to use it. This means that the one paying the endorser to advertise believes that the person endorsing the product or service is still using the product or service. The endorsement must be honest and adequately substantiated and must disclose any material connection between the advertiser and endorser [40]. With these guidelines, the dentist must take great care not to have statements of superiority or to mislead prospective patients.

In 2009, the Florida Supreme Court has ruled that a state law restricting how dentists may advertise credentials issued by bona-fide professional organizations is unconstitutional and violates the First and Fourteenth Amendments of the US Constitution [41]. The Federal District Court in California has ruled in 2010 that state laws prohibiting or restricting advertising bona fide and legitimate credentials to be unconstitutional. This ruling has set a precedent that could become the basis of further challenges in advertising of credentials in other states. Most states prohibit statements of professional superiority, advertising that is false and misleading in any material respect, and guarantees of any services [42, 43]. Since this is an area of regulation that seems to be currently under reviews and challenges, a more extended discussion of advertising in dentistry will be found in Chapter 21.

True Case 11: Dental society denial

In the early 1980s a dentist and his partner applied for membership in the local dental society and to be on the dental staff at a nearby hospital. Both the society and the hospital denied their applications due to the fact that the two dentists advertised via a public service announcement to see your dentist twice a year and promoted their location and the various services available. They appealed the decisions and requested the FTC to support their right to advertise. Upon the society's and hospital's reviews, both were accepted. (Times have certainly changed!)

Federal False Claims Act

The Federal False Claims Act applies if the Federal Government is the payer. There are also state false claims acts or health care fraud acts that apply if an insurance or state agency is the payer. The basis is to criminalize the intent to defraud the government or insurance company by knowingly and willfully providing false information or omitting information on a claim for payment for services rendered. Intent is not needed to be shown in many situations. Punishment is based on the payment received over one year and can be extrapolated to a longer period of time. Over $3000.00 is considered a felony.

It needs to be pointed out that per the Yates Memo it was suggested that corporations do not violate the false claims act but individuals do. Under this memo, you may be held liable for the false claims that are being filed with your name and information by the office you work in. Examples of violations are failure to:

1) Comply with your PPO contract
2) Take complete medical history
3) Document findings on radiographs
4) Document medical/dental necessity
5) Collect patient's co-pay or deductible.

The Federal Anti-Kickback Statute is a health care fraud and abuse statute that prohibits the exchange of remuneration, which the statute defines broadly as anything of value, for referrals of services that are payable by a federal program (Medicare/Medicaid). Violation constitutes a federal felony punishable by up to five years in prison and up to a $25,000 fine for each violation.

The Stark Law prohibits self-referral, specifically a referral by a physician/dentist of a Medicare or Medicaid patient to an entity providing designated health service if the physician/dentist (or an immediate family member) has a financial relationship with that entity.

If fraudulent billing is suspected, a profiling by the federal government or the insurance company may occur. The government or the insurance company look to the reasonableness of a claim and compares the dentist's billing patterns with other dentists. If a pattern exists of unnecessary or excessive claims for a certain procedure, the dentist may be subjected to a full practice systems review of all claims. If providing treatment beyond routine insurance covered procedures, be sure to have a signed informed consent with the patient's understanding that insurance coverage is not available for that particular procedure and they are financially responsible.

If profiled, provide information supporting your treatment and involve the patient to state that the dentist provided all the treatment that was billed. If there is a problem with the needed supporting information, change billing practices, seek legal advice, and try and negotiate a settlement. The final amount sought can be staggering as seen in True Case 12. For example:

For every routine extraction the insurance company is billed for a surgical extraction. The overpayment was $50.00 for each extraction. Upon review, the insurance company finds that it has been done for 12 years.

Claimed incorrect/contested fee $50.00

×

Rate of code usage of 40 times per week

×

Number of years enrolled in the PPO was 12 years/524 weeks

=

$1,048,000 Payment Demand

True Case 12: Fraudulent billing

A large multi-state dental corporation provided treatment for a large patient population on Medicaid. Upon review by the government of 60 patients it was found that all extractions were up-coded and billed as a surgical extraction and not a routine extraction when done. The patient chart was well written to support the up-coded surgical extraction. However, when compared to the radiograph, it should have been billed as routine. Some of the radiographs showed only an anterior tooth root tip, only in tissue, with part of it being exposed and billed for a surgical extraction with notes indicating that a periodontal flap was done, bone removed, tooth sectioned, and then removed and sutured. The expert witness/consultant also found up-coding for quadrant scaling and root planning, when charting only supported a routine prophy. Many of these cases did not even have periodontal charting done. The dental corporation settled for five million dollars.

References

1 Illinois Dental Practice Act (Ill. D.P.A.), 225 ILCS 25/Section 49.
2 California Dental Practice Act (Ca. D.P.A.), Part 1, Business and Professions Code, Division 2, Chapter 4, Article 5, Section 1706.
3 New York State (NYS), Education Law, Article 133, Section 6612.
4 Ill. D. P.A., 225 ILCS 25/Section 5.
5 Ca. D.P.A., Part 1, Business and Professions Code, Division 2, Chapter 4, Article 1, Section 1601.
6 Burton Pollack, *Law and Risk Management in Dental Practice* (Chicago, Ill.: Quintessence Publishing, 2002), p. 15.
7 Ibid., p. 37.
8 Ibid., p. 30. https://www.epa.gov/sites/production/files/2016-12/documents/dental-elg_final_fact-sheet_12-2016.pdf, accessed April 25, 2021.
9 NYS Environmental Conservation Law Section 27-0926, Subpart 374-4.2.
10 Ca. D.P.A., Part 3 California Code of Regulations, Article 1, Section 1014.1.
11 "National Practitioner Data Bank Guidebook," The Healthcare Quality Improvement Act of 1986, P.L. 99-660; Data Bank Title IV Regulations, 45 CFR Part 60; Subpart A,
12 Data Bank Title IV Regulations, 45 CFR Subtitle A (10-1-06 Edition), Part 60.
13 45 CFR. § 164.514(b)(2)(i)(R).
14 https://www.hipaajournal.com/what-are-the-penalties-for-hipaa-violations-7096, accessed May 8, 2021.
15 Telephone Consumer Protection Act 47 U.S.C. § 227, https://www.fcc.gov/sites/default/files/tcpa-rules.pdf, accessed May 30, 2021.
16 NYS Education Law, Article 133, Section 6604.
17 Karen Fox, "California OKs Portfolio Exam for Licensure," *American Dental Association News*, Vol. 41, No. 19 (2010), p. 1.
18 Ill. D.P.A., 225 ILCS 25/Section 19.
19 Ca. D.P.A., Part 1 Business and Professions Code, Article 2, Section 1635.5.
20 Ibid., Sections 1636, 1636.4, 1636.6.
21 NYS, Education Law, Article 133, Section 6604a.
22 Ca. D.P.A., Part 3 California Code of Regulations, Article 4, Section 1107.
23 Ill. D.P.A., Part 122, Section 1220.440.
24 Ca. D.P.A., Part 3 California Code of Regulations, Article 4, Section 1017.
25 Ca. D.P.A., Part 3 California Code of Regulations, Article 4, Section 1016.
26 "Nevada Board of Pharmacy Prescription Monitoring Program Information," http://bop.nv.gov/links/PMP/kh, accessed March 5, 2022.
27 Ca. D.P.A., Part 1 Business and Professions Code, Article 2.1, Section 1647.1.
28 NYS Education Law, Article 130, Section 6509.
29 NYS Rules of the Board of Regents, Part 29, Section 29.1.
30 Ca. D.P.A., Part 1 Business and Professions Code, Section 1680.
31 Ill. D.P.A., 225 ILCS 25/Section 23.
32 NYS Commissioner's Regulations, Part 61, Section 61.9.
33 Ill. D.P.A., 225 ILCS 25/Section 4.
34 Ca. D.P.A., Part 1 Business and Professions Code, Article 7, Section 1741.

35 Ca. D.P.A., Part 3 California Code of Regulations, Article 5, Section 1087.

36 NYS, Education Law, Article 133, Section 6608.

37 Ca. D.P.A., Part 1 Business and Professions Code, Article 7, Section 1753.5.

38 Joseph P. Graskemper, "Ethical Advertising in Dentistry," *Journal of the American College of Dentists*, Vol. 76, No. 1 (2009), p. 44.

39 Federal Trade Commission, Revised Endorsement and Testimonial Guide, 16 CFR Part 255.

40 Ibid.

41 *Ducoin, DDS v. Viamonte, DDS*, Florida State Surgeon General, 2nd Circuit Court, (2009).

42 NYS Regents Rules, Part 29, Unprofessional Conduct, Section 29.1.

43 Ill. D.P.A., Part 1220, Section 1220.421.

3

Definitions and Legal Concepts

It is to be hoped that you will never be involved in a dental malpractice lawsuit. Approximately one in seven dentists is sued annually. Of course, some dentists may never be sued, while others, as we saw in True Case 8, may have many lawsuits. It should be pointed out that you do not have to have done anything wrong to be sued. Keep in mind that anyone can sue anybody for anything at any time for any amount, if a lawyer can be found to take the case (usually not a difficult task). I have found that good communication with the patient helps create a solid and trusting doctor–patient relationship, from which misunderstandings leading to lawsuits may be avoided. Patient communication will be covered in Chapter 8, Chapter 22, and Chapter 7 in "Leadership and Communication in Dentistry." The doctrines, rules, and definitions discussed will provide a fundamental understanding that will help you make decisions regarding your dental practice or a possible legal case.

Negligence

Negligence is the building block of most malpractice lawsuits. Negligence is a lack of ordinary care or the failure to use reasonable care that results in harm to the patient. Malpractice is a special form of negligence. It is that negligence arising out of the doctor–patient relationship that results in an alleged malpractice lawsuit. There are acts of commission, which is the performance of an act that a reasonably prudent dentist would not have done, and there are acts of omission, which is the failure to act as a reasonably prudent dentist would have done. So, it is not only what you have done that could be found to be professional malpractice, but also what you failed to do. Hence, professional malpractice is based in the concept of negligence. There are four components to negligence that must all be met in order for the patient/plaintiff to prevail in a dental malpractice lawsuit. These components are:

1) A duty to render care must be shown.
2) A breach of that duty must have occurred.
3) The patient must have suffered damages.
4) The damages suffered by the patient must be proximately caused by the breach of that duty [1].

A "duty" arises when a dentist acts in such a way that his or her actions give rise to a risk of harm to the patient. In other words, when a dentist treats a patient or even consults a patient, the dentist has a duty to be reasonably prudent in his or her care and not to cause the patient harm. Ethically this is referred to as nonmaleficence, as will be discussed in Chapter 17. So, the duty begins when the dentist and the patient voluntarily enter into a doctor–patient relationship (to be further discussed in Chapter 4). This occurs whenever the dentist undertakes to render care, including giving

Professional Responsibility in Dentistry: A Practical Guide to Law and Ethics, Second Edition. Joseph P. Graskemper.
© 2023 John Wiley & Sons, Inc. Published 2023 by John Wiley & Sons, Inc.

professional opinions that may affect a patient's care or health care decision, thereby creating a professional relationship with a corresponding "duty to care" for the recipient patient. Therefore, when providing an opinion, even in a social setting including social media, the dentist must exercise reasonable care in giving that opinion such that the patient will not be harmed if the patient relies on that opinion.

True Case 13: Amalgam tattoo – melanoma

The patient went to the dentist for his regular maintenance visit. The patient had numerous dark round spots on his gingivae and some in the vestibule areas. The dentist was not too concerned since the spots were typical of a patient being of African descent and the patient did have numerous large amalgams on most of his posterior teeth. The dentist made notes on the appearance and locations of the spots and had even drawn a mapping of the location of the spots. He told the patient that they were most likely amalgam tattoos and not to be overly concerned about them. He informed the patient if any changes occur to let him know. Approximately a year later, the patient came in regarding a change he noticed. On examination, a very large typical example of a melanoma was present. When he asked the patient why he did not come in sooner, the patient stated he thought it would go away. The patient was properly referred, but months later the patient died. The dentist was then sued for wrongful death, misdiagnosis, and failure to refer, among other causes of action. The court found for the plaintiff because the dentist did not properly inform the patient of how to properly examine the area with a mirror and what changes to look for regarding color, size, shape, and texture of the area. The case was appealed but settled before the appeal decision.

So, when you tell a patient not to worry about that amalgam tattoo, as the dentist did in True Case 13, be very sure it is an amalgam tattoo, and not the beginning of a melanoma. Inform the patient how to look, what to look for, and to immediately inform you of any changes whatsoever. It would be wise, if your diagnosis is not 100% certain, to refer to the appropriate specialist. Here the duty was not only to inform the patient of the existence of the "amalgam tattoo," but also to inform the patient of how to look and what to look for, not just to look. You may also want to take an intra-oral photograph for future comparison and also want to take a photo with the patient's cellphone so he or she may also have a record of it and for their own comparison at later dates.

Once the dentist acts in such a way that a duty arises, he or she must fulfill that duty. You will be held to a duty to treat the patient with reasonably prudent care. In other words, you will have a duty to treat within the standard of care (to be discussed in Chapter 12) and to adhere to treatment techniques and procedure protocols. Your failure to fulfill that duty is considered a breach of duty, the second component of negligence. That duty arises when the doctor–patient relationship begins and continues until the patient or the doctor ends that relationship. The duty to properly treat the patient with reasonably prudent care covers all aspects of treatment, from opinions to actual treatment to after-treatment care.

If you have failed or breached that duty, the patient may suffer damages, the third aspect of negligence. There are three major types of damages: special damages, general damages, and punitive damages. Special damages are any out-of-pocket expenses that the patient may have had to pay in order to become whole again due to negligence that resulted in injury to the patient, including lost income. General damages are the financial compensation for pain, including but not limited to emotional, mental, and/or physical pain. Punitive damages are awarded to the plaintiff when the defendant is to be punished for his or her action or inaction [1]. These are normally not seen in dental malpractice cases. Damages have come in some very surprising areas as shown in True Case 14 and 15.

True Case 14: Divorce due to paresthesia
The patient sued the dentist for causing her husband to divorce her. The patient had an extraction of a mandibular third molar. The extraction caused a profound paresthesia of half the mandible, including her tongue and lip. She claimed that her husband divorced her because kissing and other romantic endeavors left him unfulfilled. The case was settled out of court.

True Case 15 (True Case 1 Revisited): Lawsuit due to dentist's criticism
The patient sued the dentist for miscarriage due to a failed pulpal debridement. The patient, who was four months pregnant, came into the office of a board-certified endodontist with severe pain. A radiograph was taken with double lead shields, blood pressure was taken, and informed consent was given. The dentist used 3% carbocaine to anesthetize the tooth. The tooth had a large amalgam. The dentist made a conservative opening and debrided the tooth performing a pulpotomy. The patient was to return if any further pain occurred or after the delivery of the baby. About six months later the endodontist was sued for malpractice that allegedly caused the miscarriage of the baby which prompted a claim for wrongful death. While pregnant, the patient had gone to another dentist who was going to perform a root canal. When he could not get down the canal due to some blockage, he took a radiograph and found metal-like radiopacity within the canal. He told the patient that the previous dentist had broken a file off in the canal and the tooth needed to be extracted. During the arbitration, with the use of a magnifying glass, the expert witness showed the radiopacity to be a piece of amalgam and not a separated file. The radiograph also showed that the previously existing amalgam was completely removed by the second dentist. Hence, the canal blockage was actually due to the second dentist's treatment. The case was dismissed.

Both of these true cases illustrate that unexpected damages can be claimed by the plaintiff.

If the first three elements of negligence have been met, then comes the hardest part of proving negligence. Were the damages suffered either directly or indirectly (proximately) caused by the dentist's breach of his or her duty to provide reasonably prudent care? To answer this, an expert witness is usually employed to explain whether the treatment rendered was within the standard of care, whether treatment protocols were followed, and the technical aspects of the dental treatment proximately caused the patient/plaintiff's damages. Expert witnesses for both parties will look closely to see if there is any connection between the treatment rendered or failed to be rendered and the claimed damages. Remember, the damages claimed do not have to be a direct result of treatment, as seen in the previous two cases. If you refer a patient to another health care provider whom you knew or should have known to practice below the standard of care, you may be held liable for any damages suffered by the patient as a result of the other health care provider's treatment (see Chapter 21).

Definitions

There are many legal concepts and doctrines that pertain to dentistry. Here are some of the more common concepts, definitions, and doctrines. Many will be discussed in more detail in various later chapters.

Standard of Care: The skill and care that a dentist would bring to a similar case, or that which ordinarily is used by reasonably qualified prudent dentists in similar cases and circumstances [1].

Informed Consent: The dentist has a duty to give the amount of information about the treatment that a reasonable person would want to know so an informed decision can be made.

Express Consent: The dentist and patient agree to the treatment to be rendered. It may be oral or written.

Implied Consent: When treatment is being provided and the patient permits it to continue without objection. By the inaction of the patient, the patient is consenting to the treatment.

Informed Refusal: When the patient refuses the treatment recommendations of the dentist, he or she must be informed of the risks of the decision.

Statute of Limitation: The deadline for filing a lawsuit. Lawsuits must be filed within a certain time following the event that resulted in a claim.

Exceptions to statute of limitation: Foreign Body – instruments not normally left in the body such as a part of an endodontic file, surgical instrument or even the tip of a periodontal scaler and the patient was not informed at the time it happened.

Fraudulent Concealment – Knowingly not addressing a known problem which eventually causes the patient harm such as a patient with a new crown with an open contact, telling the dentist at each recall maintenance visit about food impaction and the dentist ignores to correct it. The patient then develops a severe periodontal problem resulting in the loss of the tooth.

Fraud – Wrongful deception intended to result in financial or personal gain. The submitting fraudulent claims to a patient, third-party payer such as an insurance company or the Federal or State Social Services.

Continuing Treatment – When the dentist continues to provide treatment with no regard to the patient's complaint such as a poor fitting denture or not diagnosing periodontal disease in a timely manner, even though the dentist kept seeing the patient at six months recall maintenance visits, the dentist will be held liable for not treating that problem.

Statute of Repose: The outside limit at which a lawsuit may be filed. Not all states have this type of statute.

Res Ipsa Loquitor ("the thing speaks for itself"): The patient would not have been injured but for the dentist's negligence, and the damages are obviously due to that negligence. In such cases, an expert may not even be needed, because it is obvious to a reasonable person. The extraction of the wrong tooth that was fully intact and healthy is an example that fits this concept.

Habit and Custom: The habitual behavior or custom of the dentist to do something always in the same way is evidence that the dentist did do it. Such habitual behavior is admissible as circumstantial evidence that the habit or custom was followed on the occasion in question. It is better to record in the chart what was done as evidence of your habit or custom rather than to rely on this concept. You will need to have substantiating evidence to support your claim of habit and custom, such as the testimony of your assistant. This can be hard to do if, for example, that assistant is no longer employed, lives far away or left your employment on bad terms. The courts normally do not look favorably on habit and custom as support for the defendant dentist. If it is not in the records, it is usually viewed as not happening.

Comparative/Contributory Negligence: The actions of the patient/plaintiff may have contributed to or partially caused the injury claimed by the patient/plaintiff, such that only partial recovery for the damages claimed will be allowed. The recovery for damages is reduced by the percentage of the plaintiff's contribution to their own injury.

Respectable Minority Rule: The dentist should not incur liability merely by electing to pursue one of the several recognized courses of treatment [2].

Last Clear Chance Doctrine: If you rely on information from another health care provider that you knew or should have known to be incorrect, you may be held liable for the patient's damages, because you had the last clear chance to act properly and prevent the patient from being harmed [3].

Hold Harmless Clause: It is a release of any and all claims, actions, suits, charges, and judgments whatsoever that protects business owners and associates from being sued when someone suffers damage, bodily injury, or financial loss on business property due to the other's actions. This protects each party, the employer and the associate, of the contract from any liability incurred including to defend and indemnify each in the event of a lawsuit or alleged malpractice by the other.

Vicarious Liability: This is the indirect responsibility for another, where one person, normally a superior, is held liable for the action of another.

Respondeat Superior ("let the master answer"): This is a form of vicarious liability that applies to employer/employee relationships due to the employer benefiting from the employee's endeavors.

Hearsay Evidence Rule: Secondhand information should not be admitted as evidence.

Best Evidence Rule: Only the best evidence that is available for examination should be admitted. Instead of asking a dental assistant what the dentist said, the best evidence rule would require that the dentist directly say in testimony what he or she said.

Res Gestae Exception to Hearsay: When statements are made at the time of or immediately after the incident in question, they may be held against the person (the dentist) when that statement is not in that person's best interest. Such statements may be admitted into evidence. So be sure neither you nor any of your auxiliary personnel say "Oh no," "Oops," or any other indication that something has gone wrong.

Best Judgment Rule: The dentist must use his or her best judgment when prevailing practice is unreasonably dangerous for a particular patient [4]. For example, it is the prevailing practice to replace teeth with a removable partial denture. A normal healthy patient with numerous missing teeth may opt for a removable partial denture rather than implants. However, if the individual were handicapped in such a way that he or she was not able to remove the partial denture if it became dislodged, the patient would possibly have a high risk of the partial causing damages by becoming lodged in the throat or airway. Hence, the dentist may use his or her best judgment not to fabricate a removable appliance for this patient and leave the patient partially edentulous.

Errors in Judgment Doctrine: This is a very difficult doctrine to employ and is not always upheld in the dentist's favor. A dentist should not be held liable for the patient's damages if reasonable, non-negligent care and proper diligence were used [5]. There must not be a total disregard of the patient's well-being. For example, a patient requires the replacement of missing teeth, the span of which is just a little bit longer than ideal. The patient, after a long discussion of treatment options, opts to have a long span bridge that is just over the limit of Ante's Rule (one and a half times the replaced root surfaces is needed in the abutment root surfaces to properly support the fixed bridge). The root surfaces of the abutment teeth for this patient appear on radiographs to be very healthy and larger than normal. The crown–root ratios are within normal limits. After a full, honest, informed consent discussion, the patient – understanding all the risks involved – exercises his autonomy and still opts to have the long span bridge. When the bridge fails, the dentist may cite this doctrine in his defense. Of course, it would have been better for the dentist to refuse to do the bridge from the very beginning.

Damages: The financial compensation for the injury due to another's wrongful act.

Special Damages: This is the monetary amount to cover the patient/plaintiff's out-of-pocket expenses, which would include but not limited to, the dentist's received fees, subsequent treatment needed, future needed treatment, lost wages, and transportation.

General Damages: This is the monetary amount given to the plaintiff for their mental, physical and emotional pain and suffering.

Punitive Damages: This is rarely granted in dental malpractice cases. Its intent is to punish the defendant for bad acts. True Case 16 shows that continualy ignoring the patient's problem, sometimes called "watchful neglect", can result in a bad law suit.

True Case 16: Tennessee case Tolliver v. Gamble

The dentist fabricated a full upper denture. The patient returned many times to have the denture adjusted. The dentist kept telling the patient that she would get used to it. The patient was never satisfied with the fit of the denture. After several years of adjustments, the patient sought legal recourse. The court found that the dentist ignored the continued complaints of the patient which the court found to be a total disregard for the patient and awarded the patient $150,000 in punitive damages.

Discovery Rule: The Statute of Limitations begins when the patient discovers or should have discovered that the alleged injury occurred as a result of the treatment that had been rendered.

Occurrence Rule: The Statute of Limitations begins when the alleged injury (negligent treatment) occurred.

Battery: The unlawful touching of another.

Assault: A threatened or attempted physical attack by someone who appears to be able to cause bodily harm if not stopped.

Assault and battery charges have been filed against dentists when an informed consent was not given by the patient.

References

1 Joseph Graskemper, "A New Perspective on Dental Malpractice," *Journal of the American Dental Association*, Vol. 133 (June 2002), p. 752.

2 Joseph H. King, *The Law of Medical Malpractice in a Nutshell* (St. Paul, MN: West Publishing, 1986), p. 66.

3 Graskemper, "A New Perspective on Dental Malpractice," p. 753.

4 King, *Law of Medical Malpractice*, p. 72.

5 Ibid., p. 71.

Part II

The Practice of Dentistry

4

The Doctor–Patient Relationship

The beginning of the doctor–patient relationship is when a professional duty attaches to the opinions and actions of the doctor. The basis of this relationship is in contract law. Contract law has three elements that must be fulfilled: the offer, the acceptance, and the consideration.

Basis for Relationship

The offer is a proposal to enter into an agreement. The offer must describe the intent of the offer. In other words, it must describe the intentions of the person making the offer. In a doctor–patient relationship, the intention of the doctor is to provide services. It must have certain and definite terms. The doctor offers to provide services for an ailment in return for consideration, that which the person accepting the offer will give to the doctor for the services rendered. And it must be made to the person who can accept the offer. Making an offer to a person not able to accept the offer is meaningless. One of the building blocks of informed consent is based in contract law, as will be seen in Chapter 8.

The acceptance is the voluntary act of accepting the offer. It must not be coerced or made under duress. The person accepting the offer must have the authority to accept it and must have an understanding of what is contained within the offer. As you can see, the offer and acceptance is basically a type of informed consent discussion (as is discussed in Chapter 8). Once there is an agreement by both parties as to what the contract entails, it is called a "meeting of the minds."

The consideration is the bargained-for exchange. It may include an act, a forbearance to act, or a promise to act. That act may include an exchange of money, goods, or services. For example, a patient may pay personally or through an insurance policy, provide the doctor with a service such as landscaping for the doctor's office, or bring the doctor food as seen in True Case 17. Without consideration, the offer becomes a gift to the person accepting the offer. Even if you decide to provide your services as a gift, you may still be sued for malpractice. Although your intentions were honorable to not charge the patient, you must still provide treatment within the standard of care. Being a nice person and helping another out, which most often happens when someone is in pain, does not preclude you from being sued.

True Case 17: Food for fillings

A dentist had an office in a rural area. It was not uncommon for him to be brought a pig or vegetables in payment for his dental services. It was not something that he did often, but when the patient was not able to pay with money, the goods provided were welcomed.

Professional Responsibility in Dentistry: A Practical Guide to Law and Ethics, Second Edition. Joseph P. Graskemper.
© 2023 John Wiley & Sons, Inc. Published 2023 by John Wiley & Sons, Inc.

Fiduciary Duty

Due to the fact that as a doctor with higher understanding and learned skills than the patient regarding their dental health, the patient must put some level of trust in the doctor that the doctor places the patient's best interests ahead of the doctor's interest. Fiduciary duty is placed on a person in a position of authority whom the law obligates to act solely on behalf of the person he or she represents and in good faith.

Therefore, the doctor has a legal fiduciary duty to promoting the patient's well-being. This can also be understood ethically as the principle of beneficence. (Discussed in Chapter 17.)

There are two types of contracts: express and implied. The express contract may be made orally or in writing. It is when the parties involved have a distinct, explicit, and understandable agreement as to what each party must do per the contract. An express contract must also be a direct, positive, and unequivocal agreement. Preferably, the contract should be in writing that includes all the terms of the agreement to prevent miscommunication and/or misunderstanding. The implied contract occurs when the actions or the conduct of the parties involved implies that the consideration has been mutually agreed upon. Many times, through the actions of one person, another may rely on those actions as an assent to proceed with treatment with the expectation of consideration (payment). The first person may not now say he or she did not agree. Implied contracts prevent unjust enrichment of the person who receives a service and then says he or she did not want it after the fact. For example, a patient may have an examination, be informed of the need for a crown, make several appointments (breaking the first appointment and rescheduling it), come in and sit in the operatory chair, open his or her mouth, get numb, have a tooth prepared, and have impressions taken and the crown cemented, only to say, "I never agreed to pay for it" (see True Case 27). In this situation, the patient was well aware of the treatment and made no objections when the treatment was provided. All of the signs, actions, or inactions of the patient gave rise to the presumption that the patient implied in fact to agree to the contract and receive treatment. Nothing needs to be said about the fee since the patient's actions or inactions, including silence during the procedure, implies that there was an agreement to pay for the services rendered. Nevertheless, we will see in later discussion that it is best to have proposed treatment and fees discussed and agreed to by the patient. It should also be noted that there is also an implied consent in law that exists. It is rarely used in dentistry, since it is based on an emergency situation in which there is no mutual assent to the treatment but a reasonable person would have agreed to the services rendered under the similar circumstances. These types of circumstances are usually seen in emergency medical treatment involving life and death (see Chapter 8).

In doctor–patient relationships, doctors often try to prevent a lawsuit by having the patient sign an exculpatory clause. Exculpatory clauses, being an agreement not to sue for any future negligence, have been found to be invalid, because they are contrary to public policy. In other words, signing this clause would be bad for the public in that it would allow negligent treatment to be provided and not have any repercussions. Patients would be injured without any means to address or seek reimbursement for their damages due to malpractice.

Types of Realtionships

There are four different models of the doctor–patient relationship. The guild model is based in the belief that the dentist has the expertise to treat the patient who does not have the ability to understand enough to make proper dental decisions. The agent model is based on the patient having the knowledge and understanding to properly use the dentist's expertise. The dentist becomes an agent of the patient to provide services that fulfill the patient's needs or desires. The commercial model is based on the belief that the dentist is simply a manufacturer or seller of products to the patient. Each party, the dentist and the patient, may make any agreement desirable to both parties as is based purely in contracts and not address the ethical and professional concerns of the doctor and patient. The interactive model is based on a mutually respectful relationship with equal commitments to proper, ethical, health care decision-making [1].

I refer to the ultimate doctor–patient relationship as a co-diagnosis, in which both parties contribute to the decision-making process through communication (Chapter 22). As will be discussed further in Chapter 14, communication is the basis of a healthy doctor–patient relationship and a great risk management tool. It is also discussed in Section 2, Part 1 in "Leadership and Communication in Dentistry."

When Does It Begin

Now, with the basis of the doctor–patient relationship understood, when does this relationship actually begin? The doctor–patient relationship begins when the dentist agrees and provides a service or an opinion on which the patient reasonably relies. It does not start when a patient walks into your office. The patient may walk into your office, fill out all the appropriate informational forms, and hand them to the receptionist. At which time the patient asked if the office takes his or her insurance. When told that the office does not participate with that insurance as a contracted provider, the patient walks out. There was no doctor–patient relationship established because no opinion was given. However, because personal health information was given to the receptionist the doctor is still liable for safeguarding that information under HIPAA laws, rules and regulations. This is in contrast to the "curbside" advice often given in a social setting or in a late-night telephone call. Suppose a patient or even a nonpatient comes up to you at a social gathering and asks what you think of sensitivity and a very seldom ache on a lower tooth and jaw. If you tell them that it's nothing and not to worry, and that person ends up two days later having a serious infection or heart attack; you could be held liable, because the person relied on your opinion and did not seek the needed treatment. This same scenario can be found in teledentistry (if not documented properly), Facebook or other social media communications including e-mails and texts, that give an opinion that the patient would reasonably rely upon. This is commonly referred to as a cyber doctor–patient relationship and carries the same legal liabilities as if you actually saw patient.

The question is "whether a patient knowingly seeks a physician's services and the physician knowingly accepts the patient." (Kundert v Ill. Valley Comm. Hosp Ill App Ct 3rd Dist., 2012) The court went on to state that the physician must take some affirmative action to diagnose or treat the patient in order for the relationship to exist. Giving an opinion that the patient relies upon is considered diagnosis and treatment.

Duties of Doctor and Patient

Once the doctor–patient relationship has been established, there are implied duties placed on each of the parties involved, both the doctor and the patient. The implied duties of the dentist are:

1) To be properly licensed and to fulfill the legal requirements necessary to provide his or her services to the public.

2) To use reasonable care in providing services within the standard of care (as will be discussed later).
3) To employ and to supervise employees.
4) Not to exceed the scope of expertise as qualified or authorized.
5) To make appropriate referrals.
6) To properly inform patients of treatment and outcomes.
7) To maintain patient confidentiality.
8) To complete treatment in a timely manner.
9) To not use experimental procedures without being properly informed.
10) To make the patient's records available.
11) To provide emergency care when needed.
12) To not abandon the patient [2].

But what about the patient? Patients also have some duties, though not as many. The implied duties of patients include:

1) To follow home-care instructions and keep appointments.
2) To cooperate in treatment.
3) To answer questions honestly.
4) To inform the dentist of any change in health status.
5) To pay bills in a reasonable manner [3].

These implied rights of each party to the doctor–patient relationship (contract) are based in ethics and law, to facilitate the professional flow of information and mutual cooperation for successful treatment outcomes for the patient as well as the doctor. Without these implied rights, the element of trust in the doctor–patient relationship would be lacking and the relationship would cease to exist as it does today.

Patient Relationships

Attention should also be given to possible personal relationship with a patient. Personal relationships with patients are troublesome due to the fact that one of the persons in the relationship may feel coerced. The mere claim of sexual harassment, whether true or not, are not covered by your malpractice insurance in the defense of such an allegation. Charges of sexual harassment can be elevated into criminal offenses as rape and sexual assault.

A mere hug or pat on the back may be taken as harassment. With social media communication very prevalent, care must be taken that even a LOL may be taken wrongly. Is that Laugh Out Loud or Lots of Love? You should also refrain from tasteless jokes or flirtatious banter with patients.

ADA Code 2 (G) states that the dentist should avoid interpersonal relationship that could impair their professional judgment or risk exploiting the confidence placed in them by a patient. This should be applied to the family members of patients due to the close connection with the patient. It is suggested in such a situation there should be a cooling off period of approximately two years or terminate the doctor – patient relationship.

To properly maintain a trusting, legal doctor–patient relationship, you should avoid using patients for financial gain outside of dental care, such as fundraising, donation solicitation, intrusive political and religious donations, etc. Also, you should avoid gifts that seek preferential treatment or attention. It is hard not to accept a patient's thankful gift when appropriate. To accept a patient's small thankful gift that is well within appropriateness of a doctor–patient relationship is acceptable.

When Does It End

Once the doctor–patient relationship has begun, when does it end? It may end in several different scenarios. It is obvious that the relationship will end when treatment has ended and/or the
patient goes to another dentist, as well as when there is a mutual ending of the relationship
such as a referral to another dentist better suited to treat the patient (for more on referrals, see
Chapters 21 and 24). If the doctor or the patient dies, or if the dentist terminates, sells, or trans-
fers his or her practice, the relationship also ends. For the dentist to end the doctor–patient
relationship unilaterally, a letter of patient termination (see Chapter 11) must be written to
properly inform the patient that the relationship has ended. Under contract law, if either party,
the dentist or the patient, breaches the contract, the doctor–patient relationship also ends. To
breach the contract for services, either the dentist failed to perform the services agreed upon or
the patient failed to pay or accept the services. The patient's failure to pay for the services, as
shown in True Case 18, does not release the doctor from liability for any treatment or opinion
that was rendered to the patient. Non-payment does not release the doctor from a malpractice
lawsuit.

True Case 18: No pay, no crown

The patient came into the dentist's office to have a porcelain to metal crown placed on #8
due to it being fractured. Because it is difficult to match the shade of a single maxillary
central, the crown was sent to the lab for custom shading. At the cementation appointment
the patient was not happy with the shade. Again, custom shading and staining were done
and a bisque bake (unglazed) crown was shown to the patient, who was then satisfied. The
crown was then sent for glazing. The patient failed to show for any appointments for over
three months and failed to make complete payment. When the case was taken to small
claims to collect the monies owed, it was found in favor of the patient on the grounds that
the goods (PFM crown) were never delivered. The judge did not accept the argument that
the patient would not come to have it cemented or that it was custom made. Though not the
best ruling, it was a ruling nonetheless. Nevertheless, the doctor–patient relationship was
terminated due to the patient not showing up for appointments nor paying in full for the
services rendered.

At any time that the doctor–patient relationship ends, a chart entry and/or letter informing
the patient is necessary to prevent any miscommunication that would lead to patient
abandonment.

References

1 David Ozar and David Sokol, *Dental Ethics at Chairside* (Washington, DC: Georgetown University
Press, 2002), p. 44–52.
2 Burton Pollack, *Law and Risk Management in Dental Practice* (Chicago, IL: Quintessence Books,
2002), p. 48.
3 Ibid., p. 49.

5

May You Refuse to Treat?

There is no duty to treat a patient. The duty to treat a patient arises out of the initial development of the doctor–patient relationship, as discussed previously. Every dentist has the right to treat those patients he or she chooses. However, that choice must not be based on color, creed, race, religion, national origin, or disability, including HIV, AIDS, or TB (inactive). Recently, for example, those with a positive COVID-19 test may be refused treatment until COVID negative or no longer having symptoms. As time passes, this also may change due to becoming less of a communicable infection causing less crippling consequences. Discrimination does not attach when referring a patient for needed treatment that is beyond one's skill level or competence. However, in a decision to refuse treatment based on treatment needs, be sure that the decision is equally based for all of one's patients and not due to some underlying bias. As was pointed out previously, employees also cannot refuse to treat a patient based on the aforementioned protected classes or groups. In the event that an employee refuses to treat such a patient, that employee must be fired or risk the effects of a lawsuit based on respondeat superior/vicarious liability.

On the other hand, employees should not be fired who have contracted HIV or AIDS. They should be reassigned and given a position without direct patient care. Of course, this is a heavy mandate for a small dental office with only three to seven employees. Therefore, following the labor laws of your state, proper legal advice should be sought in your employment decision-making.

For a health care provider with HIV/AIDS to continue to treat patients, a highly ethical decision needs to be made in regards to the patient's right to be fully informed of the risks of being treated by a HIV/AIDS health care provider. There is no requirement for a dentist to inform a patient of their health care status. Would such information affect the patient's informed consent to being treated? There are many factors to be weighed. When giving an informed consent, are patients told every conceivable risk that they may encounter, such as death due to the anesthetic injection? It has been held that patients do not need to be informed of every conceivable risk [1]. On the other hand, doesn't the dentist have a right to practice, using proper universal precautions? What about his or her legal responsibilities to support a family, to repay education and practice loans, and right to work? It has also been found that there is an extremely low risk of dentist-to-patient transmission when universal infection control precautions are employed. The case of Florida dentist Dr. Acer, in which the dentist more likely than not did not follow such precautions, was found to document a dentist-to-patient transmission of HIV/AIDS [2]. Hence, a decision must be made by the infected dentist, following ethical and/or legal guidelines, as to whether to inform the patient or to limit treatment procedures to those that are less invasive. Obviously, this is not an easy decision to make.

Professional Responsibility in Dentistry: A Practical Guide to Law and Ethics, Second Edition. Joseph P. Graskemper.
© 2023 John Wiley & Sons, Inc. Published 2023 by John Wiley & Sons, Inc.

Pandemics (COVID-19)

The pandemic of 2019 with the SARS-CoV-2, commonly called COVID-19 has brought new issues to the forefront. With world-wide travel available to most, the spread of infectious diseases can be wide and swift. Pandemics bring new issues to patient care and the interaction of the patient with the doctor and staff. With some states highly recommending and even mandating the vaccination of selected groups of citizens, doctors and patients became very cautious of each others's COVID vaccination status. This has called attention to the fact that some patients demand to know the COVID vaccination status of their dentist and his or her staff as seen in True Case 19. Likewise, some dentists and their staff demand to know the patient's status. Due to the high level of aerosols generated in most procedures, the patient's status should be known to the treating health care provider. It is the aerosol from the patient's treatment that is of concern. In the event of pandemic such as COVID-19, a questionnaire might be useful in informing the patient and the dental office of the possible risks of providing and receiving dental treatment. Due to the fact of wearing proper face masks, shields, air scrubbers/purifiers, and using direct patient HVAC by the provider, the status of the provider is not of much concern. Of course, the simple precaution of taking a patient's temperature upon arrival to the dental office and that of the entire dental staff each and every morning would be wise to do. The staff must understand the importance of daily temperature taking and not to report to work if having any symptoms. There have even been cases of doctors not providing the patient care unless vaccinated or tested within 2–3 days of treatment to safeguard the other patients, doctor, staff, and their families. This however should not replace the precaution of taking the patient's temperature upon arrival to the office. A patient may be refused treatment due to having a temperature, has recently traveled to a "hot spot," has recently been exposed or living with a COVID-positive person, or experiencing symptoms of possibly having a pandemic sickness. As will most viruses, mutations occur and their lethal threat usually diminishes over time.

True Case 19: Patient demand

With the outbreak of COVID-19 and vaccinations being available, the patient asked the status of the dentist, hygienist, and rest of the staff before making an appointment. When the dentist informed the patient that due to HIPAA, he cannot release an employee's vaccination status, the patient sent a very long email about the dentist being unprofessional, uncaring, and would not be returning to the office ever.

References

1 Joseph P. Graskemper, "Informed Consent: A Stepping Stone in Risk Management," *Compendium*, Vol. 26, No. 4 (April 2005), p. 288.
2 Centers for Disease Control, *Morbidity and Mortality Weekly Report*, Vol. 39, No. 29 (July 27, 1990), pp. 489–493.

6

The Medical–Dental History

By all legal and ethical standards and practice protocols, it is extremely important to have a proper and complete medical–dental history. Every time you see a patient, this history is relied on to guide you in questions such as type of anesthetic, how the patient withstands treatment, and medical complications. Therefore, the history must be complete for every patient, and an initial blood pressure must be taken. Both must be updated yearly or as needed per the patient's medical condition and the treatment to be rendered. The history must be signed and dated by the patient or legal guardian, and reviewed and signed or initialed by the dentist. At the end of the health/ medical history, the patient should sign a simple statement such as: "I hereby acknowledge the medical history is correct and complete and will inform of any future changes." The history should contain, but not be limited to, the following:

1) Past dental history, including any current problems.
2) Complete medical history and medicinal allergies.
3) Food/metal sensitivities or allergies.
4) Any prescription medications taken.
5) Any over-the-counter medications taken.
6) Any food, vitamin, or herbal supplements taken.

Many times patients do not think taking a small pill such as a baby aspirin (81 mg) is important enough to be marked down on the medical history. Additionally, a successful joint replacement without any complications many years ago may seem to be unnecessary information for a patient going to get his or her teeth cleaned. Therefore, with proper questioning, certain medical conditions requiring premedication or other precautions will be uncovered and treated accordingly.

Even though the patient has completed the health history, without investigative questioning, important facets of the patient's history may be missed, as seen in True Case 20.

True Case 20: Only Boniva

A long-term patient and friend of the dentist fractured a tooth to the extent of its being non-restorable. The patient was asked if there were any changes in her health history prior to the tooth being extracted. The patient said, "No." The extraction occurred without any complication. When the patient called two weeks later and said that the area was not healing, she was told to return to the office for examination of the extraction site. It indeed was not healing properly.

Professional Responsibility in Dentistry: A Practical Guide to Law and Ethics, Second Edition. Joseph P. Graskemper.
© 2023 John Wiley & Sons, Inc. Published 2023 by John Wiley & Sons, Inc.

True Case 20 (Continued)

The patient was again asked if there were any changes in her health that she failed to mention prior to the extraction. She then stated that she was taking Boniva, a bisphosphonate, and she felt the dentist did not need to know that information due to the fact that it helped make her bones stronger and had nothing to do with her mouth. The area eventually healed, but the patient discontinued seeing the dentist and never returned because she thought the dentist was too upset with her regarding the nondisclosure of vital information. If the extraction site did not heal properly, would the patient have been more understanding of the dentist's concern or would she have sued him for professional malpractice?

Some of the common errors are:

1) Failure to learn more about the patient's food or drug allergies and their interactions.
2) Failure to discover a medical condition (diabetes, artificial joints, arrhythmias).
3) Failure to discover temporomandibular joint (TMJ) problems (accentuated during or after a long dental appointment or a traumatic surgical procedure).
4) Failure to discover anesthetic sensitivities or reactions.
5) Failure to discover periodontal problems.
6) Failure to discover a cancer problem [1].

Therefore, the dentist should not wholly rely on a simple "yes" and "no" questionnaire. Questions requiring more than a simple "yes" or "no" should be used to clarify any questionable health history.

Other Needed Information

Other information should also be contained in the health history to help in an emergency or to gather more information such as a medical clearance, if needed, from the patient's physician. The entire staff should be attentive to the patient upon his or her arrival. For example, an elderly frail male patient walks very slowly and a little off balance. The staff notices that he is taking a very long time to fill out the forms. When he hands the forms to the receptionist, she notices that there are no medications, no health issues, and he states he can't remember his physician's name and number. When specifically asked if he has had any medical issues, he states that he recently had a heart valve replacement. Hence, the name, address, and phone number of the patient's physician must be obtained as well as the name and relationship of parent, guardian, or caregiver, if someone other than the patient fills out the forms. Besides the patient's personal information (name, address, etc.) there should also be an area for a brief description of the patient's main concern. There should be no blank lines and the questionnaire must be completely filled out (all yes and no questions answered). It is highly preferable to use a black pen because it copies well. It is very hard for an expert witness to decipher a poor copy. It is in your best interests that your chart entries are legible, to be most effective in your defense. There must also be a statement, as was previously mentioned, that the patient/legal guardian must sign that states that he or she acknowledges the health history is correct and complete. There should also be a general consent to treatment. This does not replace an informed consent for a particular procedure; rather, it is a consent that authorizes the dentist to provide dental care for the patient. An example of such a consent is, "The undersigned hereby authorizes the doctor to perform any and all forms of treatment, medication, and therapy (with patient's prior consent) that may be indicated in connection with (name of patient) and further authorizes and consents that the doctor choose and employ such assistance as he deems fit. I also understand that dental treatment and the use of anesthetic agents embodies certain risks. I have been afforded the opportunity to ask any questions."

Remember, many patients do not report aspirin or other over-the-counter drugs, vitamins, herbal supplements, other health additives, or even surgical procedures, because they believe it does not pertain to their teeth. True Case 21 shows that some patients may not even consider heart surgery a contributory factor to providing dental care.

True Case 21: Only heart surgery

A patient reported for an appointment to have a scaling and root planning performed. She was to be given local anesthetic. She lives outside the country for half the year but receives dental treatment in the United States. It is the normal procedure for the office to review the medical history with the patient at each visit, by asking if there have been any changes. The patient told the hygienist that there had been no changes. The hygienist placed a topical anesthetic on the selected areas and proceeded to get the dentist to anesthetize the left side of the mouth for the scaling and root planing. When the dentist came in and greeted the patient, asking her how her visit home to England was, she said it was terrible since she had to have open heart surgery a couple of months ago. No mention of this was made to the hygienist because the patient felt it wasn't important! The lesson learned here is that it never hurts to repeat a question to a patient, even if you sound redundant.

Therefore, you must always ask the patient or legal guardian if there are any changes at each appointment, prior to treatment.

Barriers

Many times there are barriers to allowing a valid, complete, truthful medical–dental history. Hearing, sight, and/or language may erect a barrier to the dentist in extracting needed information. These barriers are easily overcome by finding proper assistance in gathering such information. It may be cost-prohibitive for a small dental practice to provide such assistance as needed; nonetheless, there must be communication. Most times patients with such needs are aware that proper care can be provided only if they are able to communicate the problem properly. Such patients should be advised to bring the assistance needed if they have not already done so. When a patient brings someone with them, make note of the person and his or her relationship to the patient, since you are relying on this person to transfer or translate the information correctly.

Reference

1 Burton Pollack, *Law and Risk Management in Dental Practice* (Chicago, Ill.: Quintessence Publishing, 2002), p. 125.

7

Patient Abuse

Child abuse has been defined as the act or the failure to act that causes physical or mental injury, sexual abuse, or negligent treatment/emotional harm of a child under 18 years of age by a person responsible for the child's welfare under circumstances which might indicate that the child's health or welfare is harmed or threatened.

It has been found that more than 65% of all cases of physical abuse involve injuries to the head, neck, or mouth [1]. Therefore, dentists are in a prime position to be an observer of child abuse, which occurs at all socioeconomic levels. However, dentists have made less than 1% of all reports [2]. That the reporting is so low could be due to any of the following reasons:

1) The family is well known to the dental office as a "good" family.
2) There is a fear of losing good patients.
3) There is a fear of embarrassment.
4) There is a fear of reprisals.
5) The dentist may not be aware of the legal duty to report or may be afraid of the process.

Dentists are in a strategic position to recognize mistreated children. While the detection of dental care neglect is an obvious responsibility for dentists, other types of child abuse and neglect also may present themselves in the dental office. The characteristics and diagnostic findings of physical abuse (nonaccidental trauma), sexual abuse, failure to thrive (nutritional neglect), intentional drugging or poisoning, Munchausen's syndrome by proxy, health care neglect, safety neglect, emotional abuse, and physical neglect all should be familiar to the dentist.

Definitions

Child abuse is an act of commission. It is nonaccidental injury or trauma inflicted on a minor (under 18 years of age) by a parent or other caregiver. It is the infliction of serious physical injury, the creation of a substantial risk of serious injury, or commission of an act of sexual abuse against the child.

Child maltreatment and child neglect are acts of omission. Child maltreatment refers to the quality of care given the child. This occurs when the parent or caregiver fails to exercise the minimum degree of care for the child by providing food, clothing, shelter, or education. It also

Professional Responsibility in Dentistry: A Practical Guide to Law and Ethics, Second Edition. Joseph P. Graskemper.
© 2023 John Wiley & Sons, Inc. Published 2023 by John Wiley & Sons, Inc.

includes emotional abuse or neglect. Child neglect is the failure to properly provide for the child's basic needs, care, support, or health, including abandonment.

The American Academy of Pediatric Dentistry has defined dental neglect as the willful failure to seek treatment when treatment is necessary to allow for oral health with adequate function without pain and infection. This includes failure to seek treatment for untreated, rampant caries, trauma, pain, infection, or bleeding. It also includes failure of the parents to follow through with treatment once they have been informed that the mentioned conditions exist [3]. The American Dental Association (ADA) Principles of Ethics and Code of Professional Conduct states, "Dentists shall be obliged to become familiar with the peri-oral signs of child abuse and to report suspected cases to the proper authorities" [4]. The courts have even stated that a dentist who fails to identify and report suspected child abuse is guilty of professional negligence [5].

Reporting Child Abuse

All 50 states have passed child abuse reporting laws under the Child Abuse Prevention Act of 1974 [3]. These reporting laws list dentists as a mandated reporter; hence, dentists are required to report suspected cases of child abuse and neglect. Mandated reporters are protected by law from criminal and civil liabilities arising from good faith reporting of suspected child abuse. Many states have criminal penalties for failing to report a suspected child abuse case. Such liabilities are not normally covered by professional malpractice insurance. Therefore, it is wise to report any suspected child abuse case. It is better for the well-being of the child to error in your suspicions rather than overlook the abuse due to the aforementioned reasons. Ethically, with adherence to nonmaleficence and beneficence, it is the right thing to do.

To report a suspected child abuse case, most states have an 800 number you can call. You do not have to be absolutely certain of abuse to report it. Only a reasonably good faith reason to suspect that the child has been abused due to neglect or nonaccidental injury is necessary to proceed with a child abuse report.

In your patient records, do not include your suspicion of child abuse. Keep it factual with your findings reported just like any other examination notes, if it is within the normal dental exam. If suspicious marks are seen outside the head and neck areas or beyond a dentist's normal examination, you should, on separate paper, record your suspicions and physical findings, as your personal notes and not part of the patient record. Do not question the child, parent, or guardian regarding your suspicions. Do not investigate yourself. Call and report the suspected abuse to the proper authorities. Let them proceed from there. These personal notes should be kept in a separate area and not in the patient's record. In this way, the notes will be protected from the parents or caregiver when and if the child's records are requested.

In 2009, a mother was charged with dental neglect of her son after failing to follow through on the dentist's recommendation, failing to show for appointments, and eventually causing the son to be admitted to the hospital with severe infection. True Case 22 was approximately 23 years prior. Hence there has been advancement in the understanding that dental neglect is a serious offense.

True Case 22: Child neglect
In 1986, a dentist, a specialist in orthodontics, examined a new patient for possible braces. Upon examination, he found rampant caries and advised the mother that the child needed to see a general or pedodontic dentist as soon as possible for the needed dental treatment prior to any orthodontic treatment. The mother told the dentist that until the child stops eating so much candy and starts brushing his teeth more, she was not going to waste her time and money on fixing the child's teeth only to have them rot again. The orthodontist was astonished at the mother's response and again tried to explain the needed restorative dentistry. The mother became very adamant in her stance. It was a clear case of child neglect by not providing proper dental care for the child, especially when costs were not the preventive factor. The orthodontist called the Child Protective Services department in his city to report the suspected child abuse/neglect case. After describing the case to the agency, he was thanked and told that it would be put on the list; however, there were presently a number of cases of broken bones, cigarette burns, and child beatings that were currently being investigated. In other words, "We'll get to it when we can, if we ever actually do."

In a situation such as that presented earlier, ethical responsibilities set in when the cost of dental treatment makes the restorative dentistry prohibitive due to the parent or guardian's finances. If the dentist is not willing to take on a charity situation in providing the needed treatment at reduced fees or at no charge, then he or she must refer the parent or guardian to a reduced fee dental service provider, such as Medicaid, another government program, or a charitable organization.

Elder Abuse

Dentists should be aware of elder abuse because the population is aging per the National Center of Health Statistics. It was not until 2009 with the passage of the Elder Abuse Victims act that elder abuse received attention [6]. Elder abuse occurs at every socioeconomic level, across ethnic and cultural lines, within all religions and at all levels of education. In most states dentist are mandated reporters of elder abuse.

Elder abuse is a general term used to describe harmful acts toward an elderly adult, emotional or psychological abuse, sexual abuse, financial exploitation, and neglect/abandonment, including self-neglect [7]. This would include intentional drugging/poisoning, safety and physical neglect. From 2000 to 2050 it is anticipated that the percent of the population 65 years and over will increase substantially. Between 2000 and 2050, the percent of the population 65 to 74 years of age will increase by 7–9 percent. By 2040, the population 75 years and over will exceed the population 65 to 74 years of age [8].

The American Dental Association (ADA) adopted a policy in 1996 regarding abuse and neglect; it states that policy in the ADA Principles of Ethics and Code of Professional Conduct:

SUBSECTION 3.E. ABUSE AND NEGLECT. Dentists shall be obliged to become familiar with the signs of abuse and neglect and to report suspected cases to the proper authorities, consistent with state laws.

ADVISORY OPINION 3.E.1. REPORTING ABUSE AND NEGLECT. The public and the profession are best served by dentists who are familiar with identifying the signs of abuse and neglect and knowledgeable about the appropriate intervention resources for all populations. A dentist's ethical obligation to identify and report the signs of abuse and neglect is, at a minimum, to be consistent with a dentist's legal obligation in the jurisdiction where the dentist practices. Dentists, therefore, are ethically obliged to identify and report suspected cases of abuse and neglect to the same extent as they are legally obliged to do so in the jurisdiction where they practice. Dentists have a concurrent ethical obligation to respect an adult patient's right to self-determination and confidentiality and to promote the welfare of all patients. Care should be exercised to respect the wishes of an adult patient who asks that a suspected case of abuse and/or neglect not be reported, where such a report is not mandated by law. With the patient's permission, other possible solutions may be sought. Dentists should be aware that jurisdictional laws vary in their definitions of abuse and neglect, in their reporting requirements, and the extent to which immunity is granted to good faith reporters. The variances may raise potential legal and other risks that should be considered, while keeping in mind the duty to put the welfare of the patient first. Therefore, a dentist's ethical obligation to identify and report suspected cases of abuse and neglect can vary from one jurisdiction to another. Dentists are ethically obligated to keep current their knowledge of both identifying abuse and neglect and reporting it in the jurisdiction(s) where they practice [9].

In 2017, the World Health Organization stated the defined elder abuse as: A single, or repeated act, or lack of appropriate action, occurring within any relationship where there is an expectation of trust, which cases harm or distress to an older person whether or not it is intended.

Signs of Abuse

The signs of abuse are slightly different but with some similarity to child abuse. Dentists should be aware of the following signs or changes in appearance and or mannerisms as their patients age and begin to be taken care of by others. Some of these signs but not limited to are:

Lip trauma.
Ill-fitting dentures, lack of dental care, and poor dental and personal hygiene.
Fractured or unexplained missing teeth.
Broken eyeglasses or frames.
Unpaid dental bills.
Signs of being restrained (rope marks).
Elder patient statements of being physically abuse.

Reporting elder abuse is very similar to child abuse as stated earlier.

Failure to Report Patient Abuse

The failure to report varies greatly by state jurisdictions. Depending on your state law, failure to report elder or child abuse may range from a misdemeanor, fines, liability for proximate damages, to loss of license and/or malpractice insurance coverage. Some states attached civil liability to such situations.

Make sure your office staff is educated and aware of patient abuse. The dentist being a mandated reporter should be made aware of patient abuse the staff may suspect or observe.

Domestic Partner Abuse

Besides the signs of abuse already mentioned there are additional possible signs of domestic partner abuse that are not easily seen but more of a psychological sort. Be aware when the domineering partner always is present in the operatory and always speaks for the patient. The patient never speaks up or makes any decision without the other domineering partner's permission. This is only mentioned to help dentists and their staffs to be aware of these situations. If you have very strong feelings and want to help, there are two questions you may ask the patient:

Is it safe to go home?
Do you want me to contact help?

References

1 Lynn Mouden and Donald Bross, "Legal Issues Affecting Dentistry's Role in Preventing Child Abuse and Neglect," *Journal of the American Dental Association*, Vol. 126 (August 1995), p. 1173.
2 Ibid.
3 Steven W. Kairys, MD, MPH, et al., "Joint Statement of the American Academy of Pediatrics and the American Academy of Pediatric Dentistry," *Pediatrics*, Vol. 104, No. 2 (August 1999), pp. 348–350.
4 Mouden and Bross, "Legal Issues," p. 1177.
5 Ibid., p. 1178.
6 Joseph P. Graskemper, "ElderAbuse: Time for Dentist to Be Aware," *Oral Health* (May 2013), p. 14.
7 Toshio Tatraaph and M. A. Kusmekus, "National Center on Elder Abuse," Elder Abuse Information SeriesNo.1, Wahingto DC 1996, p. 1.
8 United States Department of Health and Human Services, National Center for Health Statistics, "United States 2004," DHHS Pub.No.2004-1232 (DHHS, Washinton DC 2004), p 21.
9 American Dental Associationi Principles of Ethics and Profesional Conduct – Section 3.

8

Informed Consent

Informed consent involves the conversation between the dentist and the patient prior to treatment regarding the alternatives/options, risks, benefits, and costs of the treatments discussed. Informed consent is required by law and should be documented. It is the protection of the patient's rights to self-determination in accepting or rejecting the proposed treatment. This, in turn, ethically keeps patient autonomy intact. The written form that the patient signs prior to treatment is not the informed consent. It is a documentation or memorialization of the conversation regarding the treatment that took place. Without an informed consent, the dentist may be held accountable for assault and battery, which may not be covered by malpractice insurance.

Informed consent is all about communication with the patient. Communication leads to education, which leads to knowledge, which leads to good decision-making, which leads to proper patient care, which leads to a successful office/career.

What Needs to Be Done

The dentist has a duty to give enough information to the patient to allow the patient to make an informed decision. How much is enough? And what kind of information is sufficient?

There are two standards that are prevalent: the professional community standard and the reasonable person standard.

The professional community standard states that the dentist needs to give the same amount of information that dentists in the same community are giving to their patients. This standard is slowly being replaced by the reasonable person standard due to the fact that if all the community practitioners practice below the standard of care by not properly informing their patients regarding a certain procedure, pockets of substandard care would exist. Additionally, more patients are educated and can understand the treatment and the options being offered. With easy access to information on the Internet, patients have become more knowledgeable. Therefore, it does not matter what others in the dental community are saying to their patients regarding informed consent. What matters is that enough information was told to the patient such that the patient could make an informed decision. And having such information, would a reasonably prudent person undergo the procedure knowing what the patient knew? Hence, it is called the reasonable person standard.

There are two parts to informed consent: the information part and the consent part.

Professional Responsibility in Dentistry: A Practical Guide to Law and Ethics, Second Edition. Joseph P. Graskemper.
© 2023 John Wiley & Sons, Inc. Published 2023 by John Wiley & Sons, Inc.

The information part consists of six elements that must be told to the patient for an informed decision to be made:

1) The procedure in understandable terms.
2) Reasons for the procedure.
3) The benefits of the procedure and the anticipated outcome.
4) The risks of the procedure.
5) Any alternatives and their risks and benefits, including no treatment.
6) The costs of the procedure, as can be seen in True Case 23, and the alternatives.

True Case 23: Implants include the teeth

A patient went to her general dentist. Upon examination, the patient was in need of periodontal treatment, including surgery and extensive oral reconstruction. It was decided after much discussion that the patient may be a candidate for full extractions, placement of implants, and a fixed detachable/hybrid prosthesis for both maxillary and mandibular arches. The patient proceeded with the treatment plan. After the surgery and implant placement, the patient went back to her dentist to have the final hybrids fabricated. The dentist proceeded to inform the patient the costs of the hybrids. The patient informed the dentist that she already paid the oral surgeon for the implants and the dentist should see the oral surgeon for the money, since she was only there to have the teeth put in. She told the dentist that she would have never had all her teeth taken out if it was going to cost so much. The dentist lost in this case due to not fully informing the patient of the cost of the treatment, which would have caused the patient to decide on a different path of treatment.

Due to the outcome of this case and others, be sure to tell the patient the cost of each procedure. It is the patient's right to decide on whether to proceed with the treatment, seek an alternative, or not to treat at all. Always be sure to also enter into the record that the patient has accepted or refused the recommended treatment. An easy way to document is RBAC (risks, benefits, alternatives, and cost) or BARNC (benefits, alternatives, risks, no treatment and cost) discussed and consent signed.

Information Needed

There are some situations that need not be explained to the patient. Risks that are too commonly known to the reasonable person or too remotely possible need not be told to the patient. Keep in mind that the informed consent is patient- and treatment-specific. In other words, the information given to a parent for an extraction of a loose deciduous tooth on their child and the information for an extraction given to an elderly female patient with a highly atrophied mandible and who takes a bisphosphonate medication would be different. You do not need to inform a normally healthy patient of the risk of possible death from local anesthetic because of the extreme rarity. Nor do you need to inform a normally reasonable patient of soreness after a routine extraction, because a reasonable person would have already known. It is advised to inform the patient of all directly related and reasonably foreseeable risks. The patient may waive his or her consent by assuring the dentist to proceed regardless of the risks or the patient may indicate that he or she does not want to be informed. These two situations should raise a red flag to the dentist. The dentist should fully record the patient's wishes or even possibly refuse treatment, if the malpractice risks are too high. These are one of the many "setups" that occur in dental malpractice. The "patient setups" will usually be something similar to:

> "Whatever you say, you're the doctor."
> "You are such a good dentist; I trust you to do what is right."
> "You don't have to tell me; I've had this done before."
> "Just do the best you can, I trust you."
> (Doctor setups will be discussed in Chapter 12.)

Informed consent should also apply to a pandemic situation such as COVID-19. Patients should be informed of what measures you and your staff are taking to decrease and attempt to eliminate aerosols in the office. The dentist and staff want to know what exposure the patient is bringing into the office prior to treatment. Therefore, a pandemic information consent should be presented to the patient and signed.

If obtaining consent is not reasonable, such as when a patient is under any type of sedation and requiring additional treatment or in the case of an emergency, it is not needed. However, be aware that extending treatment far beyond and not connected to the treatment agreed upon prior to sedation may not be covered. Hence, prior to any sedation, be sure to cover all possible changes to the planned treatment that may need to be addressed.

The final situation that may relieve the dentist of obtaining an informed consent is usually hard to come across in a normal dental setting. Consent is not needed if the doctor is using reasonable discretion and reasonably believes that disclosure of the risks would adversely and substantially affect the patient's condition. In a normal dental setting, we do not normally see such fragile patients, to whom revealing their dental needs would cause adverse effects. In the case of an emergency, consent is not needed if the delay in obtaining consent would result in substantial risk of further injury or even loss of life.

Consent

The consent part is composed of eight elements:

1) The consent must be freely given and voluntary.
2) The patient must be given an opportunity to ask questions and have them answered competently and completely.
3) To be informative and understandable, the information part as well as the consent part must be in a language the patient understands. If necessary, provide an interpreter or have the patient bring an interpreter with him or her to the dental appointment. If an interpreter is being used, record the name and relationship to the patient.
4) The person giving the consent must be authorized to make such decisions.
5) Consent must be obtained by the dentist or trained auxiliary personnel (per your state regulations).
6) The dentist must be available to answer any patient questions.
7) Some states require the consent to be a signed, written document for certain procedures. It is highly advisable to obtain a signed written consent for any endodontic, surgical, or other invasive procedure.
8) Consent must not be rushed or coerced.

The use of consent forms that are signed by the patient is a good risk management tool. There are also consent videos that present to the patient the information about the procedure. Whether it is a form to read or a video to watch, it does not replace the discussion that must take place for a valid informed consent. If a form or video is used, it should be tailored to the procedure being done, especially for invasive procedures such as endodontic and periodontic procedures, oral surgery, and implants. Not only should the form or the acknowledgment of watching the video be signed by the patient/guardian, but it should also be signed by the dentist and a witness (such as a dental assistant). It should also be noted in the chart that the document was signed or the video watched. The written consent should not be a "laundry list" of the risks of the proposed treatment. If such a list is used, it is highly advised to add "but not limited to" at the beginning of such a list, because you can never really foretell the future (Murphy's law).

Not every patient has the authority to consent to treatment. Who may consent to treatment may differ in some states. However, for most states, a proper consent may be given by a patient of sound mind and 18 years of age or older or by the legal guardian of the patient. Grandparents and older siblings are not legal guardians. For persons caring for a minor or a patient without full decision-making abilities, a medical authorization signed by the parent or legal guardian must be obtained. In the case of foster parents, a signed medical authorization from the state is necessary. A medical authorization should have the patient's name, a statement authorizing medical/dental care, and the name of the person being authorized to make health care decisions, and should be dated and signed by the parent or legal guardian. Sometimes, especially when the patient is in his or her late teens, is able to drive, and is under 18, further authorization of treatment or informed consent may be required. A telephone call may be relied on if a good-faith effort has been made to establish that the person granting the consent is so authorized and if the conversation is well documented. Following a good-faith effort, beneficence and nonmaleficence should ethically guide the decision to treat the patient, because it may not be in the patient's best interest to temporize or to delay treatment. Many times, as shown in True Case 24, the minor is brought to the office by one parent stating that the other parent will pay for all needed dental care via a divorce agreement. The dentist should not become involved in divorce situations. A sound policy is that the parent who accompanies the minor is the one responsible.

True Case 24: Signed consent? Forgery

A divorced patient brought in a child for needed dental care. She produced a letter signed by the father stating that he would be responsible for payment. The letter and signature looked real. After treatment and request for payment from the father, the letter was found to be a forgery. The father was upset; he wanted the child to see his own dentist since he, not the mother, was granted guardianship. The child was only visiting the mother at that time; she eventually paid.

Hence, even with a good-faith effort, problems may prevail.

Competency

How do you tell if someone is of a "sound mind" and has the autonomy to make health care decisions? There are five categories of the human capacity for autonomous decision-making.

1) Does the patient have the ability to understand the relationship of cause and effect? This is the lowest level of ability to make a decision. (A simplified example is brushing and flossing teeth helps to keep teeth and gums healthy.)

2) Does the patient have the ability to see alternative courses of action available and be able to choose one? (For example, to brush manually or to use an electric/sonic brush.)
3) Does the patient have the ability to see him or herself as one who can choose one of the courses of action? (The patient is able to choose one.)
4) Does the patient have the ability to reasonably compare the different courses of action and reach a moral judgment? (The patient is able decide which is better for him or her.)
5) Does the patient have the ability to form and choose values, principles of conduct, and personal ideals to guide his or her moral judgments, shape his or her moral reflections, and conduct him- or herself accordingly? (The patient actually goes and buys the brush and uses it to improve his or her oral health.) [1]

These five categories, although simplified by the examples, should help to guide you in your decision or determination as to whether the patient has the ability to make an autonomous decision that affects his or her health care. There will be times in your professional career when the patient meets all criteria for making an informed decision, but you will still question if the patient is of "sound mind." The final question that must be answered is, "Does the patient's perceived incapacity compromise his or her decision-making?"

To incorporate these into an autonomous informed consent to allow chairside autonomous decisions, the dentist needs to ask the following four questions:

1) Does the patient understand the proposed recommended treatment? (The treatment.)
2) Does the patient understand the possible treatment options, results, and differences? Positive, negative, and no treatment? (The risks, benefits, and alternatives.)
3) Does the patient understand how his or her decision personally affects him- or herself? (The risks, benefits, and responsibilities to him- or herself.)
4) Does the patient understand the responsibilities that attach to his or her decision and how it may affect others? (The effect on the patient's life.)

True Case 25: Two for one

A new patient, a 60-year-old male, came into the dentist office to have a bridge made from #28–30 because he lost his old one. All was normal until the dentist removed the impression and was about to cement on the temporary bridge. The patient stated that he would prefer not have it cemented because that way he can remove it and clean the teeth better. After a long discussion, the dentist was able to temporarily cement the temporary bridge. The patient explained that his old bridge was never cemented 10 years ago so he could clean the supporting teeth. The only reason he lost the other bridge is because he got seasick on a fishing trip. The patient then asked if two bridges could be made so that in the event that he lost the new bridge he would have a replacement. This occurred before HIPAA, so the dentist called the individual on the patient information sheet in case of an emergency, the patient's daughter, to check the "sound mind" of this patient. After the dentist told her about the unusual request, she said that her father had full mental capacity The dentist proceeded to fabricate two bridges. Upon delivery, the two bridges were checked clinically and the patient was again informed of the risks involved and signed the chart indicating his understanding.

If the patient appears to be inebriated or drug disabled, a valid consent cannot be had. Evaluate your patients as to their sobriety or mental capacity to grant a valid consent. If their capacity in questionable, you must inform the patient that he or she must reschedule the appointment and why he or she needs to reschedule. Even when the mental capacity may be questionable as in True Case 25, the dentist made a good faith effort to establish the patient's abllity to understand and give a proper informed consent.

Exceptions

There are exceptions to being 18 years of age for a proper informed consent. Those under 18 may give their informed consent if they are any of the following:

1) Emancipated
2) Married
3) A parent
4) In an emergency (life or death) situation
5) Pregnant.

However, the consent obtained must be based on the good-faith effort of the dentist to ascertain that the patient was under 18 and eligible to grant the consent.

Many states have laws that dictate the disclosure or nondisclosure of medical–dental history to the parent and/or guardian. New York's Public Health Law, Section 18, allows for a waiver of the confidentiality only if it benefits treatment. However, it also states that:

1) A child over the age of 12 may deny the parent/guardian access to the medical/dental information.
2) The dentist may not disclose medical information if the disclosure will substantially harm the child–parent or doctor–patient relationship or other relationships, as seen in True Case 26.
3) You may not disclose information that was given to you under the condition that the information would remain confidential.
4) You may not disclose information concerning the treatment of a minor for venereal disease or an abortion [2].

True Case 26: Teenage pregnancy

The patient, who was 17 years old, went to the dental office for a restoration. The patient's parents were well known by the dentist. Since it had been a few months since the last visit, the dentist asked the patient if there were any changes in her medical history. The patient stated that she was now pregnant. The dentist asked the patient the name of her physician, in order to properly request medical clearance for dental anesthesia and treatment. The patient stated that she did not have an obstetrician/gynecologist and had not told her parents yet. The dentist told the patient that he could not proceed without medical clearance. She asked what she should tell her parents when she informs them that the dentist could not perform the required work. The dentist suggested that she have a long talk with her parents.

Types of Consent

As discussed in Chapter 4, as with contracts, there are two types of consent: express and implied. Express consent may be oral or written, though preferably it is written. It must be understandable, direct, positive, and unequivocal, and it must pertain to the treatment being rendered. A treatment plan or financial agreement is not an express consent to the treatment. It is a financial agreement defining terms of payment. It is highly advised, and in some states required to have an express consent for any invasive procedure, such as root canal therapy or oral, periodontal, or implant surgery.

Implied consent is two-pronged: by law and by action. Implied consent by law exists when treatment is provided at the scene of an accident. Under such situations, the reasonable person would grant consent for treatment needed to save his or her life or to reduce injury. Most states have Good Samaritan laws that prevent the injured person from suing the person helping who acted in good faith. There must be no expectation of payment for services rendered by the person helping. Good Samaritan laws guard against legal claims of ordinary negligence. However, they do not protect against claims of gross negligence that is the wanton disregard of reasonable care. Implied consent by action, as seen in True Case 27, exists when the patient is aware of the treatment needed and makes no objection when the procedure begins. Hence, the consent is given by the signs or signals, actions or inactions by the patient that allow the dentist to presume in good faith that the patient actually consents to treatment.

To avoid confusion with express and implied contracts, a contract is an agreement between two parties, while the consent is the willingness/acceptance of an act, or invasion of an interest will take place. Consent is contained in and part of most agreements/contracts.

True Case 27: Lawyer threatens: write off patient's balance or be sued

The patient came into the dental office for an examination and prophylaxis. Upon examination, the dentist found that several restorations were needed. The patient scheduled an appointment and then called the day before to reschedule. This was done several times before the patient actually came in for the restorations. After the restorations were completed, the patient informed the receptionist that she would pay the balance of the bill after her insurance company paid its share. The patient was then subsequently billed for the outstanding balance, or patient portion of the bill. After several billing cycles, phone calls, and a letter asking for payment, the dentist received a letter from an attorney stating that the dentist performed treatment on the patient to which she did not consent. The lawyer stated that if the dentist would not pursue payment from the patient, he would gladly drop the pending lawsuit. The amount in question was under $500. The dentist told the attorney that the patient rescheduled three times for the same treatment and cannot now claim that she was unaware of the performed treatment. The attorney stated that he understood the situation but that the patient stood by her statement. The dentist needed not only to make a legal decision but also a risk management and practice management/business decision. Even though the dentist was in the right, it was decided that to fight the pending lawsuit would be too costly for the benefit received. Closing the office for a day of depositions, having the involvement of the malpractice insurance company, and the mental and emotional stress of a lawsuit was not worth $500. The dentist wrote off the balance only after receiving a Release of Liability (to be covered in Chapter 11).

Along with an implied consent discussion, there must be mention of what happens when the patient refuses the recommended treatment or refuses to be referred to a specialist. Often, a patient may want to exercise his or her autonomy or right to determine his or her own treatment and to not consent to the recommended treatment. As previously discussed, a patient must be informed of the risks of not consenting to the treatment. The informed consent then transforms into an informed refusal. The dentist must then inform the patient of the risks and consequences of the patient's decision not to follow the dentist's recommendations. It is highly recommended, as in the case of an express written consent, that the informed refusal has written documentation of the patient's understanding and acknowledgment. The written informed refusal should have the same format as the informed consent, stating that the patient has been informed of all the risks and having the patient and a witness sign. Situations that may arise in the dental office include a patient not wanting radiographs during an examination, not wanting a restoration of a fractured or carious tooth, or refusing to be referred to a specialist for a variety of reasons. Chapter 26 exhibits some examples of informed consent and refusal to treatment forms.

References

1 David Ozar and David Sokol, *Dental Ethics at Chairside* (Washington, DC: Georgetown University Press, 2002), p. 117.
2 New York Public Health, Title 2, Section 18, Access to Patient Information, Part 3c.

9

Records

Patient dental records are legal documents. They are a factual representation of the patient's dental treatments, diagnostics, correspondence, and consultations. It is a means of communication between dentists, a basis for doctor–patient communication clarity, and provides clear recall of past treatment information. They must be accurate, meaningful, and factual. If they are handwritten, they must be legible, otherwise they are meaningless. The patient's treatment records should contain information that would allow another dentist or an expert witness, if needed, to understand the treatment provided and the manner in which it was performed. It should also contain any pertinent information relative to the treatment being provided. Many offices have gone paperless in the last decade, with more to follow in the future. However, there are still some offices that still use paper records for a variety of reasons. Expert witnesses must rely on the legibility and retrievability of the record to be helpful in the case of an alleged malpractice lawsuit. The 14th of almost 30 record-keeping errors in the American Dental Association (ADA) survey mentioned herewith was "records not legible."

A survey done by the ADA that covered the time between 1999 and 2003 found, from the 15 dental malpractice insurance companies surveyed, that the top six record-keeping errors were:

1) Treatment plan is not recorded.
2) Health history is not clearly documented or upgraded regularly.
3) Informed consent is not documented.
4) Informed refusal is not documented.
5) Assessment of patient is incompletely documented.
6) Words, symbols, or abbreviations are ambiguous [1].

It is permissible to use abbreviations that are commonly used in dentistry. To use your own personal shorthand abbreviations within the paper or computerized chart, which would be hard for another dentist or expert witness to decipher or have no meaning at all, would be an injustice to you and your patient. As shown in True Case 28, the dentist failed to make complete proper documentation in the patient's chart regarding treatment rendered.

True Case 28: $300,000 Night Guard
A mandibular bruxism appliance was fabricated for a patient to be worn nightly. The patient returned numerous times for adjustments. The patient complained of developing bilateral TMJ

Professional Responsibility in Dentistry: A Practical Guide to Law and Ethics, Second Edition. Joseph P. Graskemper.
© 2023 John Wiley & Sons, Inc. Published 2023 by John Wiley & Sons, Inc.

True Case 28 (Continued)

soreness and shifting of her maxillary anterior teeth. Upon review by an expert witness, the patient's chart only indicated that "NGA" and the photos of the patient obtained after two years of treatment showed gross flaring of the maxillary anterior teeth resulting in malocclusion, bilateral TMD, and loss of teeth. The case was settled out of court for $300,000 based on poor records among other causes of action.

Record Entries

Making entries into a paper chart should be in black ink since it copies the best. Pencil is not allowed, nor is highlighter, scratch outs, transfigured letters or numbers or using white out. Also be sure to enter any "no show," "cancelled," or "came late" appointments to indicate the patient's non-cooperation and to record the patient's failure to have adequate home care or failure to follow referrals as noted in an informed refusal. This will help show comparative or contributory negligence. If a mistake is made in the record, do not white out, scratch out, or try to transfigure it. Simply draw a single line through the wrong entry and continue with the proper one. In many of the dental practice management software programs available, changes may be made up until a certain "lockout" time limit occurs. Most software "lockouts" occur automatically at the end of each month. It is very important to have this feature, because without an automatic "lockout," the records are open to possible falsification, which would make the records untrustworthy and indefensible in a malpractice lawsuit. There must also be a reliable back-up system for your records in case of hardware/software failure, needed retrievability and ransomware. If an error is discovered after the "lockout" period, make a corrected entry as soon as possible with the notation that it is a correction to a previous entry. Note it as a "late entry" (for more on this, see Chapter 14). At the end of each entry, always have the person who is making the entry, including any auxiliary personnel, initial that entry. Do not leave lines blank or pages unfilled. If this occurs, draw a line through the blank area to signify that nothing was added to that entry after the entered date. They should not contain any subjective statements or opinions regarding the patient or the treatment. Any correspondence with a malpractice attorney or your malpractice insurance company is to be kept separate from the patient's dental records.

The purposes of good dental records include:

1) Recording the health status of the patient at the time of the initial examination.
2) Recording the treatment provided to the patient.
3) Providing legal documentation on behalf of the patient, the courts, third-party payers, or the patient's heirs.
4) Providing legal documentation in the defense of legal claims made against the dentist.
5) Fulfilling the laws regulating professional services.
6) Advancing medical research.
7) Contributing to quality assessment and assurance.
8) Providing communication among health practitioners.
9) Helping identify victims of a mass disaster [2].

Records should include the following information:

1) Specifics, in detail, of the treatment provided.
2) Reactions to treatment, adverse and positive.
3) Doctor and patient comments (including complaints, resolutions, and patient noncompliance).
4) Radiographs, photographs, and 3-D scans.
5) Prescriptions.
6) Laboratory authorizations.
7) Correspondence and telephone conversations between the patient and other health care providers (including cancelled, missed appointments, failure of home care, and failure to follow referrals).
8) Consultations requested and reports.
9) Informed consent/refusal of treatment forms.
10) A drug and medication log (including any over-the-counter [OTC] drugs or supplements).
11) Financial information and agreements (separate from the treatment records).
12) Demographic information (including place of employment).
13) Medical and dental history (including periodic updates as needed per the patient's needs).
14) Waivers and authorizations.
15) Insurance information and claims submitted.
16) Contact persons in case of emergencies (including information about the primary physician).
17) Other information unique to the specific patient's needs [3].

With the use of paper charts, "sticky notes" have found their way into and onto the patient's chart. In a busy office, they are often used as reminders between staff members including the dentist. If they are not incorporated into the patient's chart and still present when a malpractice claim is made, they will be viewed as a non-completed chart and possibly used negatively against the defendant dentist's record keeping. Therefore, they should be dated, initialed and removed as soon as possible.

Photography has also expanded as a diagnostic and communicative tool in dental care. It is highly advisable that the patient gives his or her consent to any photos taken, even if it is non-identifiable. It should be noted that the Health Insurance Portability and Accountability Act (HIPAA) applies to all photographs taken, whether or not they are identifiable. The consent must be an explicit (written) consent to publish, duplicate, or send electronically with the acknowledgment that the photo may NOT be recalled due to the media used or the photo was published, duplicated, or sent such as, in a journal, article, or book.

Electronic Records

There are many advantages to having electronic health records (EHR). They require less storage and can be stored indefinitely. Some of the larger advantages of EHR are as follows:

1) Analysis of practice patterns and research activities.
2) Speed the retrieval of data and expedite billing.
3) Reduce the number of lost records and cost of storing paper records.
4) Allow for a complete set of backup records at little or no cost.
5) Expedite the transfer of data between facilities, regardless of geographic separation.
6) A proven long-term cost reducer.
7) Practice enhancers and a public relations tool [4].

Within the dental office there are also clear advantages over paper:

1) A legible record.
2) Standard of Care guidelines automatically triggered by diagnosis forces proper sequencing and needed criteria for proper patient care.
3) Electronic prescription alerts and possibly prevents both provider and pharmacist of potentially harmful drug-drug interactions or incompatibilities with the patient's physical or laboratory findings.
4) Electronic medical record systems can track ordered laboratory, diagnostic, or imaging tests, alert the provider of abnormal tests, and even notify the patient of the need, or the lack thereof, of future tests, diagnosis, or treatment.
5) Automatically confirm the date and times of all entries and keep a dated and timed log of all individuals, with password protected access, who have accessed the record and allowing for an audit trail, if needed.
6) Automatically generate patient educational materials tailored to the patient's diagnosis and treatment.
7) A well-documented, complete, and unambiguous dental record allows for a much easier and possibly successful defense of a dental malpractice claim [5].

It should also be pointed out that with EHR, there are some obvious problems:

1) high initial cost,
2) large training investment,
3) hardware crashes and breakdowns,
4) power failures,
5) software glitches,
6) sabotage of the system by disgruntled employees and hackers,
7) unauthorized access,
8) viruses, Trojan horses, ransomware,
9) reluctance of physicians to use the tightly controlled format for notes, and
10) other real and imagined problems [6].

Legally, above all, the EHR must be reliable. To be reliable it must have a "lockout" to avoid changes to the records, retrievable when needed and kept confidential. Besides having the proper firewall, it must have authorized password protected, audit trail worthy, and auto-shutdown of program within a short period of time of inactivity requiring re-entry of password to reopen. Recently there have been some cases finding that the EHR are becoming less reliable due to the ease of drop-down boxes that are repetitious and make all records read alike. This was found to be more likely than not what happened in True Case 29. It makes them suspicious to the health care auditors when looking at dental records for False Claims Act profiling.

True Case 29: Corporate greed

A large corporately owned multi-state, multi-location dental practice treating many Medicaid patients was found to violate the Federal False Claims Act. Medicaid found numerous suspicious claims which indicated all extractions were submitted as surgical extractions rather than routine and most prophylaxies were submitted as four quadrants of scaling and root planning,

---

(Continued)

True Case 29 (Continued)

some without any periodontal charting. Upon expert review of 75 cases, it was found that root tips only resting on the gingivae were submitted as surgical extractions with the computer-generated note stating the dentist "anesthetized the area, performed a flap procedure, sectioned the tooth, and sutured the area." This was the same note for all extractions regardless of location or difficulty. A similar note in the record regarding most routine prophylaxis was noted by the expert. Those 75 cases profiled were extrapolated by the number of years and number of patients the corporation had seen in their many offices. The case was settled out of court for $5,000,000!

Release of Records

There will often be an occasion where a patient requests his or her records. Prior to release of the patient's records or the information contained in them, the dentist should request a written authorization signed by the patient. Upon the receipt of the release, most states allow a certain time period in which to release that information, either by review, a summary of the records, and/or copies. You normally can charge a reasonable fee per your jurisdiction for clerical time and/or cost per copy. Be aware of minor's charts that may contain information that was meant to be held under confidence or viewed as privileged information. Also, some states like New York protect some patient health information from being released even under threat of a subpoena, such as HIV information. These types of protected information can only be released by the patient's authorization or a court order in some jurisdictions. However, you may not refuse the request in the case of inability to pay. Never give the original records to the patient or anyone else, including your malpractice attorney, unless under a court order. People tend to lose things, and, once lost, records may never be found.

To disclose the patient information without the written, patient-signed authorization would be considered a breach of confidentiality or even a breach of privileged information and a violation of HIPAA. There is a difference between these two types of information. Confidential information is information about the patient during the course of treatment, including the medical history. Privileged information is non-health care information that must not be disclosed in a court of law without the patient's permission. Any information that has been excluded by the patient in his or her written, signed authorization may be considered privileged information.

The dentist is able to disclose confidential information under three waivers to disclosure:

1) Express waiver: a patient-written authorization as discussed
2) Implied by law
   – mandated reporting of child abuse
   – mandated reporting of communicable diseases to a health agency [7]
3) Implied in fact
   – a patient-approved referral to another health care provider
   – patients in a teaching facility
   – most minors' information to the parent or legal guardian (exceptions noted).

Other exceptions in which a dentist may disclose information in a dental record without the patient's consent include:

1) Defense of a claim challenging the dentist's professional competence in a peer review process.
2) Claim for payment of fees.

3) Third-party payer relating to fees or services rendered.
4) Court order from a police or federal agency as part of a criminal investigation.
5) Identification of a dead body.
6) Reporting a legal violation of another health care professional, if the dentist reasonably believes it is necessary to disclose the information to comply with Public Health Code [8].
7) Sharing information with other health care providers for treatment purposes.
8) The transfer of patient records involved in practice transition or sale.

A valid written general release should contain the following:

1) Patient's name and identifying information.
2) Address of the health care professional or institution directed to release the information.
3) Description of the information to be released.
4) Identity of the party to be furnished the information.
5) Language authorizing release of the information.
6) Signature of the patient or authorized individual.
7) (If necessary) time period for which the release remains valid [9].

Costs associated with the release of records must be reasonable and cost-based. The fees may include labor, needed supplies, postage, and the cost of preparation of a summary/explanation with prior patient agreement (if allowed in your jurisdiction). Fees may not include the costs of verification, documentation, search and retrieval, or recouping capital spent on data storage, access, or infrastructure. However, most states, if not all, have laws that records cannot be withheld for non-payment of a service, treatment, or medically necessary product. The Health Information Technology for Economic and Clinical Health (HITECH) Act provides that only a fee equal to the labor cost can be charged for an electronic request. It also states that records must be released within 30 days of the date of request with only one extension allowed by informing the patient and giving the reason for the delay [10]. Most states have a maximum that can be charged such as New York is $.75 per page.

Texting

It is permissible to text a patient provided that it complies with the technical safeguards of the HIPAA Security Rule's minimum necessary standards. It must not contain any personal identifiers.

There are 18 Safe Harbor data elements that may contain "other identifying number, characteristic, or code".

1) Names
2) All geographic, subdivisions smaller that a state
3) Dates (other than year) directly related to the individual
4) Telephone numbers
5) Fax numbers
6) Email addresses
7) Social Security numbers
8) Medical record numbers
9) Health insurance plan beneficiary numbers
10) Account numbers

11) Certificate/license numbers
12) Vehicle identifiers and serial number including license plate
13) Device identifiers and serial number
14) Web URLs
15) Internet protocol (IP) addresses
16) Biometric identifiers (i.e., retinal scans, fingerprints, other identifiable scans)
17) Full face photos and comparable images (unique facial identifiable characteristics)
18) Any unique identifying number, characteristic, or code [11].

There are some inherent risks in texting with patients. One of the biggest unintended risk is phone auto-correction which is easily missed. Other risks include confusing abbreviated text, patient misidentification, misspellings, and incomplete orders [12].

Teledentistry

Teledentistry includes patient care and education delivery involving the exchange of clinical information and images over remote distances for dental consultation and treatment planning. There is synchronous and asynchronous teledentistry. Synchronous is a live video format which allows two-way interaction between the patient, caregiver, or provider and a provider using audio-visual telecommunication technology. Asynchronous is to store and forward the information (radiographs, scanned impression, photographs, etc.) through a secured electronic communication system to a provider who uses that information to evaluate and render an opinion outside of real-time or live video interaction. Teledentistry is to allow remote patient monitoring (RPM) to distant rural areas, improving access to oral health care, or during pandemic situations as used during the COVID-19 pandemic [13].

There are of course limitations to the use of teledentistry in providing dental treatment. It is very dependent on the quality of photos, videos, Internet transmissions and the ability of the dentist or non-dentist to properly capture the information. There are also the issues of confidentiality, copyright ownership, licensure requirements, malpractice coverage, and the formation of a cyber doctor–patient relationship. It should be noted that many states/jurisdictions require the dentist to have a license within the state they are practicing dentistry when rendering a patient treatment opinion. Malpractice insurance normally does not cover a malpractice claim when treating a patient without a license within the state where the patient is. Therefore, be sure to check the jurisdiction's laws regarding teledentistry. In the event that you rely on a teledentistry opinion such as an out of state oral radiologist's opinion and the opinion proves to be wrong, you will be held liable because that radiologist did not have a license in your jurisdiction and the oral radiologist may be held liable for practicing without a license. The patient must be made aware of the limitation of teledentistry through a thorough informed consent covering the possibility of a wrong diagnosis due to the inherent risks of transmitting such information.

HIPAA

Within the dental office HIPAA, as discussed in Chapter 2, attaches to many situations. Any release of unauthorized patient health information that reasonably identifies the patient is covered under HIPAA. This includes, but not limited, to social comments without the actual use of names, social media friendships with staff where either party makes any statements regarding the patient's health, and online reviews such as Google, Yelp, etc. All emails and electronic claims should be encrypted and secure. The emailing of radiographic images, photographs, or scans must have a patient signed authorization. HIPAA requires a six-year retention of records.

Retention of Records

The retention of records varies within each state and normally depends on the statute of limitations. Be sure to back up your records daily to the cloud, backup service, or a hard drive to be taken off premise for record security. Regardless of the individual state's statutes, retain the records as long as possible. Illinois requires dentists to maintain records 10 years [14]. New York requires the retention of records for at least six years or, if the patient is a minor, at least 6 years and 2 1/2 years after the minor reaches 18 years of age [15]. Massachusetts and California statutes of limitations run 2 1/2 years from the time the patient discovers or should have discovered the injury that resulted from the dental malpractice. Prior to properly disposing of old records, preferably shredding by a licensed shredder, be sure to check with your local attorney and your state's laws. Upon destruction of the records, be sure to get a certification of shredding for the records' time period.

Besides patient records most dentists are also individual businesses that must maintain business records. Some of these retention times are also governed by each state.

A partial list includes the following:

Accounts payable ledger	7 years
Accounts receivable ledger	7 years
Audit/accountant annual report	Permanently
Bank statements	3 years
Canceled checks	7 years
Checks for important transactions, including taxes	Permanently
Financial statements	Permanently
Income tax returns	Permanently
Personnel records (after termination)	7 years
Payroll records/time cards	7 years
Training manuals	Permanently
OSHA records	5 years
Daysheets/schedules	7 years
Patient billings and payments	7 years
Dental insurance claims, records, correspondence (EOBs)	7 years [16–20s]

As with patient records, seek proper advice from an accountant, attorney, or your professional liability insurance company regarding state and federal laws that may apply, in addition to your state dental practice act.

References

1 "ADA Council on Members Insurance and Retirement Programs," *1999–2003 Insurance Company Survey*, (2003), p. 9.
2 Burton Pollack, *Law and Risk Management in Dental Practice* (Chicago, IL.: Quintessence Publishing, 2002), p. 137.

3 Ibid., p. 137.

4 S. Sandy Sanbar, *Module 5 – Chapter 13 Medical Records: Paper and Electronic*, 8th Edition (Legal Medicine & Medical Ethics, 2010), pp. 1–2.

5 Ibid., p. 2

6 Ibid., p. 2

7 Ill. D.P.A. Section 1220.400.

8 Richard Weber, "Release of Dental Records," *Journal of the Michigan Dental Association*, Vol. 83, No. 6 (July/August 2001).

9 American Medical Association, Patient Confidentiality, http://ama-assn.org/ama/pub/category/print/4610html, accessed October 19, 2010.

10 https://www.hhs.gov/hipaa/for-professionals/special-topics/hitech-act-enforcement-interim-final-rule/index.html, accessed March 5, 2021.

11 Code of Federal Regulations – Title 45, Section 164.514(b)(2)(i)(R).

12 "Institute for Safe Medication Practices (ISMP)," August 2017.

13 https://www.ada.org/about/governance/current-policies/ada-policy-on-teledentistry, accessed March 13, 2022.

14 Ill. D. P.A., 225 ILCS 25/Section 50.

15 New York State, Rules of the Board of Regents, Section 29.2(a)(3).

16 "Internal Revenue Service Publication 538," *Starting a Business and Keeping Records*, January 2007.

17 John McGill, "How Long Should You Keep Your Business Records?," *Journal of Clinical Orthodontics*, (May 2003).

18 Susana Paoloski, "When Is It Safe to Pitch Office Papers?," *Journal of the Greater Houston Dental Society*, (September 2002).

19 Mark Pesavento and Elaine Pesavento, "Records Retention Schedule," *Collier, Sarner and Associates Newsletter*, Berwyn, IL, May 15, 2005.

20 Council on Dental Practice Division of Legal Affair, American Dental Association, "Dental Records", 2010. P. 25.

10

Statute of Limitations

Regardless of what state you may be in, the biggest questions that surround the statutes of limitations are: When does it start? When does it end? How long does it last? There are two basic rules that states may follow: the occurrence rule and the discovery rule. The occurrence rule allows for the statute of limitation to start when the alleged injury or malpractice occurred. New York State is an occurrence state in that the statute of limitation for malpractice is 2.5 years from the time the alleged injury occurred. New York State also has a separate statute of limitation called Lavern's Law for misdiagnosed malignancies that is a mix of discovery and occurrence rules. It is 2.5 years after the cancer was discovered and 7 years from the date of the alleged malpractice. Because the doctor–patient relationship is based on contract law, there is also a statute of limitation for breach of contract for six years. Hence, the minimal time for records retention is seven years in New York. The discovery rule allows for the statute of limitation, normally 2–3 years in such states, to start when the patient discovers or should have discovered the injury or negligence. Hence, the minimum time for records retention for a discovery state such as California allows for one year from the patient discovering the injury or within three years of the date that injury occurred, whichever comes first. There are also many variations in the different statute of limitations when minors are involved. In New York, it is within 10 years of the treatment or 2.5 years past 18 years of age, whichever comes first [1]. Per the state statute, some states empower the state dental board, as in New York's Office of Professional Discipline, to have no statute of limitation.

When to Tell the Patient

It is therefore best to inform the patient of any adverse, unexpected, or negative results of treatment as soon as possible such that the statute of limitation begins to run. It should be pointed out that the sooner the situation is brought to the attention of the patient, the more understanding the patient is likely to be, because the doctor–patient relationship is the strongest and the patient's trust is highest during treatment. If the patient discovers the situation while outside the doctor–patient relationship (perhaps from another dentist), the patient's trust is destroyed and the relationship is crushed. A bad result, not due to bad dentistry or faulty treatment, is easier to explain and better understood by the patient at the time of treatment, when the patient's trust is high. One of the principles of dental ethics is veracity – to tell the truth to the patient. Therefore, legally and ethically, the dentist's and the patient's interests are best served by the honest and truthful discussion of an adverse or unexpected result at the time it occurs. The statute of limitation will then commence.

Professional Responsibility in Dentistry: A Practical Guide to Law and Ethics, Second Edition. Joseph P. Graskemper.
© 2023 John Wiley & Sons, Inc. Published 2023 by John Wiley & Sons, Inc.

Exceptions

As with any rule, there are exceptions. The continuing treatment exception allows the patient to bring suit when the dentist continues treatment on a patient over a period of time even if the statute has run its course as seen in True Case 30 where each visit restarts the Statute of Limitiations.

True Case 30: Never fitting denture

An immediate denture had been placed and the patient had been told to wait for healing for 6–8 months. At that time, a reline was done, but the patient was still having problems. Then the dentist told the patient to "hang in there" because the dentures are new to the patient, and he continued to reassure the patient. After three years of "hanging in there" and multiple adjustments and relines, the patient became frustrated and brought a law suit claim upon the dentist. Although the denture was place over 2.5 years ago (New York statute of limitation), the patient brought suit under the "continuing treatment" exception. The statute of limitation had already run its course if taken from the first visit. The continuing treatment exception allows the statute of limitation to begin to run again at the end of the last visit even though the statute had run its course from the first visit because the treatment was continuing. The dentist lost the case with an unusual result of also having to pay punitive damages.

Dental recall notices for routine prophylaxis or periodontal maintenance have not yet been found to constitute continuing treatment. Attempts have been made to allege malpractice for not sending a maintenance/recall notification, resulting in not seeing the dentist in a timely manner and subsequently having severe periodontal disease.

The foreign body exception allows the patient to bring a lawsuit from the date of discovery or when the object should have been reasonably discovered. This applies only to objects left in the body unintendedly, such as an endodontic file. Suppose an endodontic file separates during the cleaning and shaping of the root canal. Even though many unsuccessful attempts were made to retrieve the file, the dentist decides to leave it in place, and not tell the patient. This then allows the statute to continue to run until the patient's discovery or knowledge of the file, at which point it begins to toll. Again, it is best to inform the patient at the time of an adverse outcome or event.

The fraudulent concealment exception allows the patient to bring suit when the dentist has concealed or withheld information from the patient, resulting in an injury. I often call this "flossing over" a problem. This is best shown with an example. The dentist places a crown on #14. At the six-month maintenance visit, about three months after cementation of #14, the patient mentions to the hygienist that food is always getting stuck between the crown and the tooth in front of it. Upon examination, the dentist finds an open contact between #14 and #13. Rather than remaking the crown or adding a tighter contact to an existing restoration on #13, he tells the patient to keep the area really clean by flossing it really well and mentions that he will check it again next visit. The patient comes in the next visit and neither the dentist nor the patient mentions the open contact. The dentist tells the patient all is well, even though the contact is still open. Two years later (about four years after original cementation of #14) the patient sees a periodontist in another town and is told that tooth #14 may be lost due to periodontal disease as a result of severe food impaction. Even though it has been over 2.5 years since #14 was cemented, the patient may bring a suit, under the fraudulent concealment exception, against the first dentist for concealment of the open contact by telling the patient to keep flossing it rather than correcting the problem. The statute of limitation did not begin to run until the patient's last visit or until the patient discovered the cause of the problem (depending on jurisdiction).

The statute of limitations for health care fraud may be different in your jurisdiction. At the federal level, being based on third party billing, a health care fraud claim must be filed six years after the violation. However, it allows 10 years to initiate a law suit.

Reference

1 "New York State Civil Practice Laws and Rules," Section 214.

11

Abandonment

Some cases have sought patient abandonment as a cause of action because the dentist failed to complete treatment or was not available to follow up treatment without valid legal reasons. The refusal to initiate treatment may also be seen as abandonment in certain situations where the patient has been harmed by the unnecessary delay. To avoid such a complaint, the dentist must complete the services that were agreed to and be available for patients after hours or make arrangement for coverage when away from the office [1–3].

Having the duty to complete the agreed-upon services or the duty not to withhold agreed-upon treatment does not mean you must provide treatment for free when the patient has not upheld his or her agreed-upon payment. Hence there is a difference between abandonment and severing the doctor–patient relationship. Abandonment is a disregard of the patient's well-being and below the standard of care [4]. Abandonment occurs when there is a withdrawal from treatment of a patient without giving reasonable notice or providing a competent replacement [5].

There are basically four situations in which abandonment may arise:

1) Refusal to see a patient without a valid legal reason.
2) Failure to provide proper follow-up care to rendered treatment.
3) Failure to provide proper emergency care, including after-hours care.
4) Failure to provide coverage for patient care when away from the office for extended time, such as during a vacation.

Types of Abandonment

There are two types of abandonment: Inadvertent and Constructive. Inadvertent abandonment occurs when there are mis-communications with the staff regarding appointment making, insurance coverages, refusing the patient to talk to the doctor, and poor follow up. It is not intentional. For example, the doctor mentions to the staff that he or she does not like to work on a certain patient. The staff trying to be helpful continuously give excuses to the patient whenever he or she wants to make an appointment, thereby inadvertently abandoning the patient. Constructive/intentional abandonment occurs when the doctor intends to terminate the relationship without the patient's knowledge or consent, or when it is found that the doctor failed to attend to the patient as frequently as due care in treatment would demand. In other words, failing to provide treatment in a timely manner as procedure protocols would require and/or necessitate. The failure of the patient to pay any fees is not the end of the doctor–patient relationship. End the relationship first.

Professional Responsibility in Dentistry: A Practical Guide to Law and Ethics, Second Edition. Joseph P. Graskemper.
© 2023 John Wiley & Sons, Inc. Published 2023 by John Wiley & Sons, Inc.

Avoiding Abandonment

Merely referring the patient to the nearest hospital may fulfill the legal duty to not abandon the patient in an after-hours situation. Ethically, however, it falls short of truly caring for your patient since many hospitals may not have any definitive dental care available. Nonmaleficence dictates that the dentist should cause no harm to the patient. If you are not available to patients you have treated and the patient has further injury or harm due to your unavailability, maleficence has occurred. Therefore, as discussed in Chapters 12 and 14, it is wise to telephone patients after invasive or involved treatment to prevent any claim of unavailability when a problem subsequent to treatment arises.

To avoid a finding of abandonment, the dentist should properly discontinue treatment and/or terminate the doctor–patient relationship. To properly discontinue treatment, the dentist must inform the patient that the treatment is being discontinued due to one of several reasons:

1) Not following home-care instructions such that treatment outcome is jeopardized [6].
2) Not showing up for appointments [7].
3) Not paying for services as agreed [8, 9].
4) Lying on his or her health history.
5) Unacceptable or threatening behavior, including a breakdown in the doctor–patient relationship.
6) Limiting or closing a practice.

The discontinuation of treatment does not terminate the doctor–patient relationship. The patient must still be treated for emergencies and for any treatment that would be needed to not jeopardize the patient's well-being. Treatment cannot be withheld if the patient is at a critical stage of treatment and if discontinued the patient would be harmed as seen in True Case 31. In certain situations, there may be a slowing down of treatment or providing a level of maintenance care such that the patient is given the opportunity to correct the cause for discontinuing the treatment, such as not making agreed-upon payments.

True Case 31: No Money – No Teeth

The patient was in need of complete oral rehabilitation. The dentist proceeded to prepare all the remaining teeth for crowns and bridges. The patient paid half of the fee upon preparation. When it was time for the impression, the patient stated that her husband had lost his job and she was now unable to make the next agreed upon payment. The dentist refused to treat further and told the patient to return when she has the money. A little over a year later, she returned to make payment and continue her treatment. During that year, she only had acrylic temporaries that were severely worn down and badly broken down, changing her vertical dimension The dentist took the impression, delivered the crowns and bridges without checking her vertical dimension. A few months later the patient started to complain about TMJ pain. The dentist kept adjusting the bite and made a bruxism appliance for night-time wear. The pain worsened and the patient sued the dentist. The patient won the lawsuit for just under $100,000 because the dentist did not care for the patient while waiting for payment and the temporaries should have been properly maintained.

Proper Termination

The patient must be informed of the discontinuation of treatment by certified, return-receipt-requested mail. He or she must also be informed of the conditions to begin the continuation of treatment, if the patient so desires.

The doctor–patient relationship may be severed:

1) by both parties agreeing to it,
2) when either the doctor or patient dies, or
3) when either the doctor or the patient unilaterally terminates the relationship.

There are several factors of which the patient must be informed to properly terminate the relationship and to avoid a finding of patient abandonment:

1) The date as to when the termination begins.
2) A valid reason as to why the relationship is being terminated, such as loss of trust in the relationship, numerous missed appointments, etc.
3) His or her current condition and treatment needs.
4) That emergencies will be covered for a reasonable time (possibly two weeks for a city practice and more time for a rural practice, depending on your area's demographics).
5) That you are willing to make copies and transfer records to a new dentist (you may charge reasonably for reproduction of records).
6) About your expectations of how any outstanding balance will be handled.
7) That you will give information on how to seek a new dentist (preferably refer to the local dental society rather than a specific dentist) [10].

You must not terminate the relationship if the patient is in an unstable condition. This may include leaving the patient with temporary crowns as seen in True Case 31. The dentist must continue care till the patient is safely transferred to another provider for a reasonable time per the skill and/or distance of a subsequent provider. If a group practice is involved, be sure to include the entire group of providers and practice name in the termination letter and not just the one treating the patient. It may be better to complete the procedure (e.g., deliver the crown) than risk a lawsuit of alleged abandonment. The costs and time involved to defend such a claim may dictate a practice management decision to deliver the crown and then seek payment. Proper financial agreements might have prevented such a scenario. Most state dental practice acts do not allow the dentist to refuse the transfer of records if money is owed. It should be also pointed out that to charge a patient whom you want to get out of the practice for copying records may not be the best public relations for your practice, in that bad news travels faster and wider than good news. Making the patient more upset may not be the best way to terminate the patient from the practice from a practice management viewpoint.

Be sure to note all information in the chart as well as copies of all correspondence with the patient. The patient termination should be sent via certified, return-receipt requested mail.

In many situations of terminating a patient, there will be a credit on the patient's financial account and/or the patient will request a return of fees paid. Although a dentist may not have done anything wrong, as in True Case 27, it would be best to consider all risks and benefits of refusing to return the requested amount or write off a balance. Many dentists have tried to retain the fees paid when the patient requests a refund, only to find themselves being sued upon their refusal. The amount the dentist would be sued for is usually many times greater than the amount of refund requested by the patient.

Release of All Claims/Anti-defamation Clauses

When refunding the patient's money, always retain a Release of Liability/All Claims form, signed by the patient, prior to refunding any money. The Release of Liability/All Claims form should have an antidefamation clause to prevent the patient from speaking unfavorably or posting negative comments on the Internet. A communication is defamatory if there is intent to harm the reputation of another as to lower him or her in the estimation of the community or to deter third persons from associating or dealing with him or her [11]. A Release of Liability/All Claims form will normally, although not always, prevent a lawsuit, even when the dentists makes a good effort as seen in True Case 32. The dentist is strongly advised to seek legal counsel from his or her personal attorney or to contact his or her malpractice insurance company for proper legal advice, since various jurisdictions differ on requirements of such a document.

True Case 32: Patient outsmarts dentist

A dentist received a letter from the patient requesting a refund of approximately $350. The dentist informed the patient that he would do so only if the patient would sign a Release of All Claims form. He sent the form to the patient to be signed, only to have it sent back torn in half. The patient informed the dentist that either she gets the money or she is going to a lawyer. Trying to prevent further problems, he wrote the check with a release of all claims statement on the back stating that the endorsement of this check will release the dentist of all claims. The patient cashed the check but tore off the end of the check that had the release statement. The bank processed the check even though a part was missing.

All correspondence of this sort should always be sent certified, return-receipt requested, and copies of everything should be retained. If and when a situation arises in which the dentist is unsure of what to do, contacting the malpractice insurance company, personal attorney, or the local dental society peer review (to be discussed in Chapter 13) may provide guidance.

As mentioned in Chapter 2, any money returned to a patient per the patient's written request must be reported to the National Practitioners Data Bank. In an attempt to circumvent such a reporting, it may be advised to offer the refund with the aforementioned release of liability prior to receiving a written request and to pay any refund from personal funds. Again, it is always advised to seek proper legal counsel prior to taking the situation into your own hands.

Saying you're sorry may complicate the situation to the point of being used against you if the patient claims malpractice. A good way to show understanding is to let the patient know that it is your intent for patients to feel good about the care they receive. Do not mention that you are sorry about the treatment and/or the results.

References

1 *Specht v. Gaines*, 16 SE 2nd 507.
2 *King v. Zakaria*, 634 SE 2nd 444.
3 *Johnson v. Vaughn*, 370 SW 2nd 591.

4 *Watkins v. NC State Board of Dental Examiners*, 358 NC 190 (1982).

5 *Hill v. Medlantic Health Care Group*, 933 A2nd 314 (D.C. 2007).

6 *Urrutia v. Patino*, 297 SW 512 (1927).

7 *Roberts v. Wood*, 206 F Supp 579 (1962).

8 *Goldman v. Ambro*, 512 NYS 2nd 636 (1987).

9 *Surgical Consultants, PC v. Ball*, 447 NW 2nd 676 (1989).

10 Joseph Graskemper, "A New Perspective on Dental Malpractice," *Journal of the American Dental Association*, Vol. 133 (June 2002), p. 757.

11 Black's Law Dictionary.

12

Standard of Care

The standard of care is often misused and confused with treatment techniques, parameters of treatment or practice, and procedure protocols. The standard of care is relative to patient care from the start of the doctor–patient relationship to its end. Procedure protocols and treatment techniques are relative to the performance of a procedure. The standard of care is much wider in scope than procedure protocols and treatment techniques. It is not defined as "what everyone else is doing." It is not what the specialist is doing. It is not what the dental school is teaching. It is not what the study club agrees on. It is not what the latest self-proclaimed dental guru is doing. All of these may and, more likely than not, will be practicing within the standard of care. All dentists think they are treating their patients within the standard of care. Some have attempted to define the standard of care as the best he or she can do under the circumstances or what the specialist would do under the same or similar circumstances.

These definitions do not completely define the standard of care. The definition has not changed, but how dentists practice has changed. How the standard of care is applied and interpreted evolves with the development of new materials and treatment modalities. It is made malleable by practitioners who perform successful new techniques, as well as by the treatment failures that find their way into the courts [1].

The standard of care is actually mentioned in the definition of negligence as discussed in Chapter 3. The second element of negligence is a breach of the duty to render care. Did the dentist violate the applicable standard of care? Whether the dentist provided treatment above or below the standard of care is one of the biggest stumbling blocks of a malpractice lawsuit. In other words: Did the dentist more likely than not provide treatment below the standard of care that subsequently and/or proximately caused the patient's damages?

How It Began

The first mention of a standard of care was in the case of *Vaughan v. Menlove* in 1837. The court described it as the "reasonable caution a prudent man would have exercised under such circumstances" [2]. The theory then gravitated to the health care professions. When applied to dentistry, the objective criteria judging the conduct of the defendant (dentist) needed to be changed from "a reasonable man of ordinary prudence" to a higher level for two reasons [2]. First, as members of a learned profession, dentists are expected to possess and exercise skill and knowledge beyond that of ordinary individuals. Second, as to matters involving professional skills and knowledge, the

Professional Responsibility in Dentistry: A Practical Guide to Law and Ethics, Second Edition. Joseph P. Graskemper.
© 2023 John Wiley & Sons, Inc. Published 2023 by John Wiley & Sons, Inc.

conduct of a dentist should be evaluated in terms of professional dental standards determined by the dental profession, hence the need for expert witnesses. In the late 1800s, professionals and others who undertook any work calling for special skills would be required not only to exercise reasonable care in what they do, but also to possess a minimum standard of special knowledge and ability [3]. Thus, it may not have been sufficient for the dentist to provide the best treatment he or she could, even with the utmost of good faith, if that treatment is below a minimum standard.

In 1898, the case of *Pike v. Honsinger* clearly stated the elements of the standard of care. Each of the 10 elements presented in this case has developed and evolved to its current understanding [4].

1) Possess a reasonable degree of learning and skill ordinarily possessed in the practice locality.

The locality rule or community standard states the dentist will be held to the level of treatment at which other dentists are operating in their local communities. This rule is slowly becoming watered down or replaced with the "reasonably prudent dentist standard." With the availability of information for the profession through continued education, which all states now require, and the ease of keeping up to date with technical advancements through journals and the Internet, the local community rule is being found to be too narrow in its scope. It also evolved away from the locality rule, because concerns arose regarding the reluctance of doctors to testify against one another, especially if they know the defendant and live or work in the same community. This poses the possibility of insulating and perpetuating pockets of substandard practice due to a limited availability of expert witnesses, which would be unfair to claimants. This is similar to the discussion of informed consent in Chapter 8. It also creates a possible conflict of interest for the expert witness when he or she knows the defendant.

For the most part, dentists from New York, Kansas, or Washington have equal access to the most recent advancements in dentistry. Hence the locality rule has evolved into a wider scope termed the "reasonable prudent standard." *Riley v. Wieman* (1988) stated, "We cannot accept the ... application of the 'locality rule.' ... conforming to accepted community standards of practice usually insulates (the doctors) from tort liability" [5]. It further applied the locality rule as a minimum standard and placed a further requirement that doctors use their "best judgment and whatever superior knowledge, skill, and intelligence they have" [5].

2) Use reasonable care and diligence in the exercise of skill and the application of his or her learning.

The reasonably prudent dentist standard states the dentist will be held to the level of care that a reasonably prudent practitioner would have provided under a certain set of circumstances [6].

What is reasonably prudent? *Helling v. Carey* (1974) found that the non-use of a simple procedure, although the procedure was not typically used in that community for patients under 40 years old, was below the standard of care [7]. This decision was based on the conclusion that if a simple procedure would show early signs of disease, and thereby allow an early, more successful treatment or even prevention, it should have been used. Thus, the non-use of such a procedure – because its use is not a standard within the professional community – is not a reason to limit liability. That 1974 case clearly spelled out that the standards for a procedure or treatment, as set forth by a profession, may be found to be unreasonable if the procedure is basically pain-free, easy, and inexpensive, takes little time, provides a great benefit, and was not done [8]. The procedure should have been done regardless of whether it is a standard within the professional community. Use of a periodontal probe is a good example. Using a periodontal probe routinely during examinations is a painless, quick, easy, inexpensive method to check for periodontal disease. Even if all dentists in the community do not use a periodontal probe on examinations, a dentist's non-use of the periodontal probe probably would be considered below the standard of care [9].

This concept was again stated in *Vassos v. Raussalis*: "The skill, diligence, knowledge, means and methods are not those 'ordinarily' or 'generally' or 'customarily' exercised or applied, but are those that are 'reasonably' exercised or applied. Negligence cannot be excused on the grounds that others practice the same kind of negligence" [10].

Because of the technical aspect of dentistry, a judge and jury need to rely on an expert to explain what is expected of a "reasonably prudent" dentist. It is the expert's duty to review and explain what the treatment in question should have been, had a "reasonably prudent dentist" performed the treatment. What the expert witness actually does in his or her office is not relevant, although many times that may be the same. He or she is to make the treatment in question comprehensible to the judge and jury [9]. The expert witness could be your best friend or your worst enemy. Keeping clear and concise patient records is of utmost importance for the expert to properly review the case. The expert witness testifies regarding:

1) The standard of care the dentist is held to: Was the treatment technique within the standard of care? Were all procedure protocols fulfilled?
2) Whether the dentist caused the patient's injury by the departure from the standard of care.
3) Whether the injury is permanent or temporary.
4) Whether the alleged malpractice the proximate or direct cause of the injury.
5) What treatment is needed to restore the patient to health.
6) The cost of the treatment.

For a dentist to qualify as an expert, the courts look to his or her skill, training, and experience. In *Fitzgerald v. Flynn*, the court stated, "It is the scope of the expert witness' knowledge and not the artificial classification by title that should govern the threshold of admissibility" [11].

In other words, just because someone considers him- or herself a dental specialist does not make that person an expert witness. The relevant criteria are the individual's knowledge and familiarity with the procedure in question. Therefore, a general dentist with knowledge and familiarity with a procedure may be found competent to testify as an expert witness against a specialist. For example, if a specialist fails to secure informed consent from a patient before providing treatment, a general dentist with experience in such treatment may be found to be an expert witness for or against the specialist [12]. In a 1993 case, *Daubert v. Merrell Dow Pharmaceuticals, Inc.*, the United States Supreme Court held that judges are the gatekeepers to allow only sound scientific knowledge to be admitted in court. There are five factors used to determine validity of the expert that must be fulfilled: (1) whether the theory or technique in question can be and has been tested; (2) whether it has been subjected to peer review and publication; (3) its known or potential error rate; (4) the existence and maintenance of standards controlling its operation; and (5) whether it has attracted widespread acceptance within a relevant scientific community [13]. It is not always necessary to have an expert witness as in *res ipsa loquitur* ("the thing speaks for itself") cases, such as in the extraction of the wrong tooth. There must be a lack of ordinary care on the part of the dentist, which a reasonable person, not being a dentist, would not have done.

Is the standard for the specialist dentist different from that for the general dentist? According to Prosser, the courts have held that the standard may be modified if the practitioner holds him- or herself out as having greater skill and knowledge than the general practitioner. In that case, such a practitioner probably will be held to a higher standard [12,14]. Does this become a double standard of care of local/general dentist versus national/specialist?

Conversely, consider the case of a patient who, despite receiving a referral, opts not to see a specialist but wants the general dentist to perform the procedure, perhaps because of reasons such as distance or cost. If the general dentist performs the procedure and it ends in a bad result, would he or she be held to a standard that is lower than that for a specialist (depending on state law and the specifics of the case), but not below a minimum level that the patient is entitled to receive, that is, that of a reasonably prudent dentist in the same or similar situation? [12]. It would be best for the dentist to not treat the patient if the dentist is unable to meet the acceptable minimum level of care. Hence, refusing to treat the patient may be in the patient's best interest (no harm would come to the patient). Ethically, beneficence and nonmaleficence would then be held intact.

In *Cummins v. Donley*, the court held that if the defendant (dentist) represents him- or herself as having greater skill than the minimum common skill of a reasonably prudent defendant (dentist), and the patient accepts treatment with that understanding the standard of care will be modified [15].

Again, in *Riley v. Wieman* it was stated that "a specialist may be held liable where a general practitioner may not. The resulting two-tiered standard preserves the benefits of the locality rule while compelling doctors to use available methods that may exceed local standards" [5]. The duty still remains for the dentist to be reasonably prudent and to inform the patient of the opportunity to be referred for treatment to another practitioner of greater skill [12]. In other words, as Dirty Harry said in *Magnum Force*, "A man has got to know his limits."

3) Use his or her best judgment in exercising skill and applying his or her knowledge.

The best judgment rule was stated in *Toth v. Community Hosp. at Glen Cove*: "If a physician fails to employ his expertise or best judgment ... he should not automatically be freed from liability because in fact he adhered to acceptable practices. ... A physician should use his best judgment and whatever superior knowledge, skill, and intelligence he has" [16]. Much reliance has been placed on evidence-based dentistry (EBD). To simply rely on EBD as a defense of a malpractice suit, when said EBD would not have been the best choice of treatment for a specific situation, the dentist's reliance on EBD as a defense may not be held in the dentist's favor. Every patient presents with unique needs and circumstances that may require the dentist to use their best judgment based on their knowledge, training, and experience to help the patient who may not easily fit into the EBD scenarios.

In other words, a dentist may not hide behind the fact that he or she pursued acceptable EBD treatment and then claim to be free of all liability. Conversely, if the treatment protocols call for a specific way to treat the patient but the dentist chose to treat differently in the patient's best interest, the dentist should not be held liable for using his or her best judgment. In a case wherein a dentist selects a procedure that may be in conflict with traditional treatment, but without additional risks to the patient, he or she may possibly not be held liable for using his or her best judgment in treating the patient. An example of best judgment rule is the use of cantilevered bridges when a removable partial denture would be the more conventional treatment of choice. Although cantilevered bridges are acceptable in limited circumstances, they have been found to be an unreasonable alternative when used improperly. Another example is that of patching a hole in a crown or filling in a void at the margin of a crown rather than replacing it. If the accepted procedure to replace the crown would not be in the patient's best interest due to various situations such as age, periodontal issues, or medical history, if there is no added appreciable risk to the patient by treating with a cantilevered bridge or by patching the crown, then the dentist should not be held liable, because he or she used his or her best judgment [12]. It should be noted that a complete and proper informed consent is paramount if attempting such a procedure.

4) Possess that learning and skill that is possessed by the average member of the profession and in good standing.

The use of term "average" in this context loosely means that one half of the dentists are practicing below the standard of care and one half are practicing above it. This, however, truly is not the case, because more than one half of all dentists practice above the standard of care. In the place of "average," "reasonably competent" has been accepted by the courts [17].

The Restatement of Torts stated the following: "The fallacy in the 'average' formulation has been explained as follows: [The standard of care] is not that of the most highly skilled, nor is it that of the average members of the profession ... since those who have less than ... average skill may still be competent and qualified. Half of the physicians [dentists] of America do not automatically become negligent in practicing medicine [dentistry] ... merely because their skill is less than the professional average. ... [The standard] is that which is common to those who are recognized in the profession ... itself as qualified, and competent to engage in it" [18]. Hence, having a license to practice dentistry makes you qualified and competent to practice within the standard of care.

A more practical way of looking at this element of "average" or "reasonably competent" in regard to the standard of care is to think of an egg that is divided into fourths. The top three quarters, more likely than not, fall within the standard of care. There is no line above which one practices within the standard of care or below which one does not practice within the standard of care [19]. A bad result is not necessarily outside the standard of care, if all treatment protocols have been met and all other facets of the standard of care have been fulfilled. The patient is entitled to the degree of care and skill that is expected of a reasonably competent dentist acting in the same or similar circumstances.

5) Keep abreast of developments in the field.
Keeping up with the current developments in dentistry is partially the reason why states now require dentists to earn continuing education credits. However, this does not mean that you must perform every new technique (or that which is being promoted by the latest self-professed dental guru). When adopting the new techniques, dentists must be reasonably prudent and competent in their use. Dentists must also be aware of any advancements and inform patients of newer treatment options as they develop, even if the dentist chooses not to perform the procedure him or herself. Although a dentist may not perform implant procedures – a newer procedure for some – he or she should inform the patient of the possibility of being an implant candidate and refer the patient to the proper dentist if the patient opts to receive implants [8].

6) Follow approved methods.
With the advent of adhesive restorative materials, implants, and other advances in dentistry during what I refer to as the current "Platinum Age" of dentistry – because "Titanium Age" doesn't sound as good – dentists face many choices of materials, techniques, and procedures. When selecting a less popular method or material, a dentist should not be held liable if there is a "respectable minority" using the same method or material. In *Downer v. Vielleux*, the court held that "a physician [dentist] does not incur liability merely by electing to pursue one of several recognized courses of treatment" [20]. However, what constitutes an acceptable level of support for a particular technique is yet to be determined. I believe a dual approach should be used. On one hand, if progress is to be made, standards should be broad enough to allow innovation and advancement in the treatment modalities. On the other hand, the patients should be protected from ill-considered and untested procedures [19]. It remains unclear what is to be considered a "respectable minority." In *Kelly v. Carroll* (1950), the court held that "generally recognized treatment" would suffice to include the respectable minority [21].

Leech v. Bralliar in 1967 held that 65 physicians qualify as respectable [22]. In 2000 the approved jury instructions for California stated, "Where there is more than one recognized method of diagnosis or treatment, and not one of them is used exclusively and uniformly by all practitioners of good standing, a physician is not negligent if, in exercising (his or her) best judgment, (he or she) selects one of the approved methods, which later turns out to be wrong, or not favored by certain other practitioners" [23].

The courts should consider the following factors when determining whether the respectable minority rule should be applied on a wider basis: availability, effectiveness, and safety of other treatments; the patient's having given the dentist a fully informed, written consent for the procedure; and consideration of the technical support and research available for the treatment in question. Also, the dentist should have been properly trained in such procedures and be reasonably prudent in their use.

7) Follow ordinary and reasonable care.

The standard of care does not require the dentist provide the highest possible level of care, although dentists should strive continually to improve patient care. Dentists must only provide ordinary and reasonable care in a prudent and competent manner to be within the standard of care. They may not go below the minimum level of care to which the patient is entitled. As mentioned before, if a dentist holds him- or herself as providing a higher than ordinary level of care, you may be held to a higher level of standard of care [24].

8) Give proper instruction.

The standard of care extends to the information given to patients regarding how to care for themselves after treatment. Postoperative instruction must be given after treatment because the patient may continue to need care after he or she leaves the dental office. Without proper instructions, patients may be harmed [25]. Again, ethically, nonmaleficence is held intact when fulfilling this element of the standard of care. There are many situations that may entail further home care instructions to complete the patient's care: for example, not to bite hard on a new amalgam, not to eat due to numbness, or to bite on gauze after an extraction.

As was pointed out in Chapter 11, the postoperative care also extends to vacations or other times when the dentist is unavailable. Depending on your state's dental laws, it may be legally sufficient to direct the patient to the nearest hospital when an untimely emergency arises and/or the dentist is unavailable during a vacation. Ethically, maleficence may occur when the patient delays treatment due to the emergency room not being dentally equipped or not having dental personnel on staff. Hence, the ethical concept of nonmaleficence may be breached. It is ethically best to have a fellow colleague "on call" to care for your patients when you may be unavailable.

The situation of having a colleague "on-call" while you are away is a good way to allow proper coverage when away from the office. There are problems that may arise when the referred dentist (Dr. B) is not as ethical as you (Dr. A) were led to believe. For example, the patient fractures a tooth while you are away for 10 days. The tooth was painless and only needed a core buildup and a crown. Rather than temporize or smooth the tooth, Dr. B preps the tooth for a crown and schedules the patient for a prophylaxis for determination of the proper shade, prior to cementation of the crown. Dr. B has violated a legal concept called agency. This concept makes Dr. B an agent of Dr. A such that Dr. B has a fiduciary duty to provide services to the patient with Dr. A's interest held above his own. Dr. A may have legal action against Dr. B for loss of income. This does not mean that Dr. B may not charge for emergency services rendered, but he or she should be judicious in the treatment provided. So, be sure the doctor you have "on call" is trustworthy.

9) Not offer guarantees.

Simply because a dentist tells a patient that he or she can save a tooth with endodontic therapy or periodontal surgery, it is not a guarantee that the tooth will be saved. I call a lot of the statements made by dentists "dentist setups." Statements such as "I can save that tooth," "Your smile will be perfect when I'm done," or "This will be an easy extraction" are no-win situations for the dentist. Building up the patient's expectations beyond those which the dentist is capable of providing, or building up expectations to an unattainable degree, can set up the practitioner to possibly become a defendant. However, there is an implication that the dentist will act competently and prudently to bring about a good result for the patient through ordinary and reasonable care [26]. Many state statutes and codes of ethics do not allow guarantees of treatment results.

10) Errors in judgment.
If the treatment ends in a bad result, that alone will not be a successful cause of action. The "error in judgment" is not a solely determining or ruling doctrine that determines the fate of a malpractice case. In *Fall v. White*, the court stated that "a doctor will not be negligent if he exercises such reasonable care and ordinary skill even though he mistakes a diagnosis, makes an error in judgment or fails to appreciate the seriousness of the patient's problem. There cannot be a total disregard for the patient's problem" [27]. An example may be found when a patient has discomfort in a tooth and the dentist diagnoses the need for root canal therapy, core build-up, and crown. Six months after completing treatment, properly following all treatment protocols, the patient complains that the tooth never felt good and now has pain upon biting. After multiple attempts to relieve the pain, a 3-D scan was done and the tooth is extracted only to discover a root fracture in the tooth. The dentist possibly made an error in judgment but still fulfilled the standard of care. Minimum requirements of skill and knowledge must be met regarding the diagnosis and treatment of the patient. The error in judgment relates to the choice of treatment. It does not relieve the dentist of negligence/malpractice in the performance of the chosen treatment/procedure. The dentist must proceed as a reasonably prudent and competent dentist, providing, at the very least, ordinary and reasonable care [28].

Challenges

With the recent development of expanded duties of dental assistants, dental hygienists, and mid-level dental providers, how will the standard of care be affected? Will there be various levels of the standard to attach to each level of care or will these dental auxiliaries be held to the standard of care to which the patient is entitled to and has received from dentists? Due to the predictability of most dental procedures, do patients view dentists as infallible in their treatment? In other words, if the treatment is not successful or has a resulting problem, it must have been due to the dentist not doing it right: The expected infallibility of the health care provider.

The standard of care has evolved and will continue to evolve by way of the various rulings of trial and appellate courts, advances in dental research, better continuing education programs, and the normal progression of the daily practice of dentistry. A good example is the use of 3D scanning in the placement of implants and extraction, among other uses. The standard of care is not a line above or below which dentists fall. It is the manner in which a dentist must practice. A bad result is not necessarily outside the standard of care, provided that the patient has received the minimum level of care to which he or she is entitled. This includes the proper referral to another dentist when the level of care to which the patient is entitled is beyond dentist's capability [8].

References

1 Joseph Graskemper, "The Standard of Care in Dentistry," *Journal of the American Dental Association*, Vol. 135 (October 2004), p. 1449.
2 *Vaughan v. Manlove*, 3 Bing. NC 467, 132 Eng.Rep (1837).

3 Graskemper, "Standard of Care in Dentistry," p. 1450.

4 *Pike v. Honsinger*, 155 NY 201, 49 NE 760 (1898).

5 *Riley v. Wieman*, 528 NYS 2nd 925 (1988).

6 Burton Pollack, *Law and Risk Management in Dental Practice* (Chicago, IL: Quintessence, 2002), p. 71.

7 *Helling v. Carey*, 83 Wash 2nd 514, 519 P 2nd 981 (1974).

8 Ibid.

9 Graskemper, "Standard of Care in Dentistry," p. 1451.

10 *Vassos v. Raussalis*, 658 P 2nd 1234, 1289 (1983).

11 *Fitzgerald v. Flynn*, 167 Conn. 609, 618, 356 A 2nd 887,892 (1975).

12 Graskemper, "Standard of Care in Dentistry," p. 1452.

13 *Daubert v. Merrell Dow Pharmaceuticals Inc.*, 509 U.S. 579 (1993).

14 William L. Prosser, *Handbook of the Law of Torts* (St. Paul, MN: West Publishing, 1971).

15 *Cummins v. Donley*, 11 NJ 418, 94 A 2nd 680 (1953).

16 *Toth v. Community Hospital at Glen Cove*, 528 NYS 2nd 925 (1988).

17 *Shilkret v. Annapolis Emergency Hospital Assoc.*, 276 Md 187, 349 A 2nd 245 (1975).

18 Restatement of Torts, 299 A, comment e, p. 75.

19 Graskemper, "Standard of Care in Dentistry," p. 1453.

20 *Downer v. Vielleux*, 322 A 2nd 82, 87 (1974).

21 *Kelly v. Carroll*, 219 P2d 79 (1950).

22 *Leech v. Bralliar*, 275 F Supp 897 (1967).

23 California Book of Approved Jury Instructions (BAJI), 6.03.

24 Graskemper, "Standard of Care in Dentistry," p. 1454.

25 Ibid., p. 1454.

26 Ibid., p. 1455.

27 *Fall v. White*, 449 NE 2nd 628, 635 (1983).

28 Graskemper, "Standard of Care in Dentistry," p. 1455.

13

Peer Review

When problems arise between the patient and the dentist, the dentist, if a member of organized dentistry (American Dental Association and its various state components), may suggest to the patient that submitting the problem to peer review may be the most efficient, cost-effective, and constructive option. Peer review is an impartial mechanism to resolve disputes between the patient and the dentist about appropriateness of treatment and the quality of care. Fee disputes are not a basis for a peer review due to Federal and State anti-trust laws that would view it as a control on competition based on costs/fees. As will be discussed in dentistry's social contract in Chapter 17, self- or internal discipline (which is required of a profession via its social contract) is fulfilled through the establishment of peer review.

First established in 1970 by the American Dental Association only allowed the review of radiographs and the patient records for peer review proceedings. In 1973 a civil liability exemption was accepted to prevent lawsuits when the result was not favorable. But by 1988, this exception/immunity was removed from review activities that fell under antitrust scrutiny. There have been further minor revisions as situations arose. Most jurisdictions stand in support of peer review decisions. However, it does not shield the dentist from an Office of Professional Discipline or other type of state licensure review agency. Most times though, it accepts the peer review decision. It also ends the doctor–patient relationship.

Cases not to be reviewed if in litigation or collection proceedings, alleged fraud or violation of the state's dental practice act (better to be brought up to the state board directly), dentist-to-dentist complaints (better to be brought up to the State Dental Society's Judicial or Ethics Committees), or if it is beyond the statute of limitations.

There are three types of peer review depending on your state dental society:

Mandatory – where dentists must take part and abide by the decision.
Participatory – where the dentist optionally takes part in the peer review.
Optional – where the dentist's cooperation and compliance are voluntary.

Peer review is usually initiated by a patient's complaint or by a dentist with the patient's consent. Both parties, the dentist and the patient, must sign an agreement to abide by the findings of the peer review and to agree not to sue each other. The fees or payments that relate to the complaint may be placed in an escrow account by one or both parties. The maximum amount refunded to the patient would be the fees paid for the treatment. All proceedings are confidential and the proceedings and the amount, if refunded, may not be reported to the National Practitioners Data Bank, depending on your state [1].

Professional Responsibility in Dentistry: A Practical Guide to Law and Ethics, Second Edition. Joseph P. Graskemper.
© 2023 John Wiley & Sons, Inc. Published 2023 by John Wiley & Sons, Inc.

The dentist and the patient are interviewed by a panel of dentists, which may also include a layperson. First the peer review committee will attempt to resolve the problem through mediation. If the mediation is unsuccessful, a panel of clinicians examines the patient and the dentist's records, and the committee will interview the patient and the dentist. Each group of dentists on the panel is different, to prevent any type of injustice, bias, or conflict of interests. Either party may be represented by an attorney at any time of the peer review process. Once the local peer review committee has made its decision, either party may make an appeal to the state-level peer review. If the patient has already had the disputed treatment redone, then it is not able to be reviewed, and consequently is not acceptable for peer review. Other criteria for peer review are that:

1. The complaint must involve appropriateness of care or quality of care;
2. The treatment must be within the state's statute of limitations;
3. The matter is not in litigation, or has been resolved by litigation or in the collection process;
4. The complaint has not been referred to the Office of Professional Discipline or similar state agency.

In the case of a minor, such proceedings are pursuant to the various state laws that must be observed. Peer review decisions, depending on the jurisdiction, may shield the dentist from a lawsuit. Some states, at the trial court level, may uphold the decisions of the peer review as final. Depending on your jurisdiction, the result of the peer review may not need to be reported to your malpractice insurance company [2]. If the dentist does not agree with the result of a local peer review, the dentist may appeal to the state level peer review, which must be based on a procedural error or there are new facts that have been discovered as seen in True Case 33.

True Case 33: Peer review

A dentist completed a three-unit bridge (#20–#18) on a patient, who was a well-known local television news anchor. The patient was shown the bridge prior to cementation so the aesthetic quality could be approved. The patient agreed to its shade and the bridge was cemented. After approximately two months (two billing cycles), final payment had not yet been received. The office called the patient and informed that the color was wrong and that another dentist was in the process of making a new one. It was suggested to the patient to contact the peer review prior to removal of the old bridge. The local peer review decided in favor of the patient, even though the patient had approved the shade, had the bridge removed prior to peer review and had pointed out his dislike of it only when a request for payment was made. The dentist requested an appeal due to the fact that the bridge had been removed not allowing for clinical review, and the local news anchor made it known that a TV news story would show how local dentists cover up for each other. The dentist won on appeal to the state-level peer review, and the patient paid the amount due without any news story appearing on TV.

References

1 ADA Council on Dental Benefits, *Peer Review in Focus*, 2010, p. 42.
2 Ibid., p. 32.

14

Risk Management

Risk management has evolved as litigation against dentists has increased since the 1970s. In 2005 the American Dental Association (ADA) produced a survey of 15 dental malpractice insurance companies that covered 104,557 dentists regarding the incidence and severity of dental professional liability claims between 1999 and 2003. The incidence of claims and the severity of claims actually diminished. The top three areas involved in paid claims for adverse outcomes for general dentists were:

1) Corrective dental treatment needed, including implant treatment (30.7%).
2) Failed root canal (14.3%).
3) Parathesia/nerve injury (8.3%) [1].

The procedures that had the most failure cases (currently there has been a large rise in implant-failure cases) were:

1) Crown and bridge, including implant cases (21.8%).
2) Root canal treatment (20.0%).
3) Simple extractions (13.6%) [2].

Hence, in many cases, the claimed maltreatment was reversible or able to be retreated.
   As to the allegations made which involved a paid claim, there were:

1) Failure to diagnose (12.3%)
2) Inappropriate procedure (11.7%)
3) Failure to obtain informed consent (8.5%)
4) Failure to refer (5.4%).

More than half of the paid claims were under $10,000 [3].
   As the number of malpractice lawsuits against dentists increased in the 1970s, risk management courses began to arise under the banner of "better records to provide a better defense." It was often proclaimed: "Records, records, records." The next development was dentists being sued for not properly informing the patient. The mantra then became: "Inform before you perform." With the progression of risk management from properly completing records to obtaining proper informed consent, the current level of risk management includes the inclusion of the patient in a discussion that allows the patient to be able to take part in his or her treatment plan's decision-making process [4]. I refer to this as a "co-diagnosis" (see Chapter 23).

Professional Responsibility in Dentistry: A Practical Guide to Law and Ethics, Second Edition. Joseph P. Graskemper.
© 2023 John Wiley & Sons, Inc. Published 2023 by John Wiley & Sons, Inc.

All these developments in risk management, from records to informed consent to the actual inclusion of the patient in the decision-making process, are important to prevent an alleged malpractice lawsuit. Other current views include "treat your patients as your friends," "a value-centered practice," and "make your patients part of your dental team," though risk management has now evolved to a new proactive perspective: practice enhancement through risk management [5].

Before further discussion of risk management, basic knowledge, and the dos and don'ts of risk management, be sure to understand the difference between an incident and a claim as described in Chapter 1. True Case 34 shows the possible result of reporting too many incidents that may occur when not attempting to reach a reasonable mutual solution.

If you truly believe the problem is only an incident that is easily corrected without a patient's legal threat, then try and work out a solution agreeable with the patient. As the saying goes, "The secret of life isn't what happens to you, but what you do with what happens to you." When confronted by an upset patient, there are several key guidelines you should follow. First, make sure you understand the patient's problem: what he or she is actually angry about. Be very attentive and listen. Then look at it from the patient's point of view: be understanding and empathic, not sympathetic; don't try to placate the patient. Have confidence in what you are saying and stay calm at all times. Ask the patient, "How can I make you happy?" Then work toward a positive solution for both of you. Keep in mind that an alleged malpractice lawsuit, even if it is found in your favor, will be emotionally, physically, and financially draining. However, be alert to the legal ramifications of returning the patient's money, paying another health care provider, or redoing treatment for free. Each of these situations may return to haunt you. If a basic mutual understanding of how the problem will be resolved is agreed upon, be sure to do it properly. If not executed with care, it may appear to be an admission of wrongdoing (malpractice) in the eyes of the patient and his or her attorney. Recently, some states such as Ohio have ruled that the showing of empathy/regret to the patient for an unanticipated, adverse outcome is not admissible at trial. Before you say you're sorry, check you jurisdiction and/or malpractice insurance carrier for advice. In such cases, guidance from your malpractice carrier may be worth their involvement.

True Case 34: Too many "near misses"

The dentist who graduated dental school approximately five years earlier had several incidents where patients made complaints about several different treatments, including removable partial denture, complete denture, a root canal, and surgical postoperative infection. Over those past five years he had contacted the insurance carrier regarding how to handle these incidents. All situations were eventually treated, corrected, or satisfied without any malpractice claim. When it came time to renew the dentist's malpractice insurance, he was told that it could not be renewed at the same rate. Either he would have to pay an additional premium or he would be refused coverage due to the fact that he reported, in their opinion, too many incidents. This led the insurance company to think that he had a problem in his patient communications or in the treatment he was providing. The dentist retained coverage elsewhere.

The Dos and Don'ts of Risk Management

1) *Do retain your records as long as possible* (see Chapter 8). Do not ever give original records or radiographs to anyone, including your attorney or insurance company, unless under a court subpoena.

   Having been involved in many defense and plaintiff attorney offices, I usually see one or two unmarked, unnamed small radiographs floating around or even on the floor. With today's digital radiographs, retrieval is much easier unless they have been deleted. Prior to any radiograph deletion (if storage/backup can no longer accommodate), be sure to print out several copies and mark them as final copies. No deletion should be made prior to the time while the statute of limitation runs its course. It would be best to electronically archive and not delete the old digital images, if possible.

   If you are employed, make certain the employer retains the records for at least 10 years after you leave and that you have the right to have access to those records if needed. If you are selling your practice, be sure the buyer retains the records at least 10 years after the sale and that you have access rights to those records if needed.

   Both of these situations are necessary with employment or buy/sell contracts so you can have access to needed records in the case of an alleged malpractice lawsuit. Without such agreements the other party may not allow you access without a court subpoena or may even destroy the old records.

2) *Do document all cancelled appointments, late arrivals, and no-shows along with any reasons given.* Do document the patient's failure to cooperate with your care, including home care instructions. Both of these documentations allow and support the defense's argument of contributory negligence, as described in Chapter 3. They also provide reasons to terminate the doctor–patient relationship, if necessary, as discussed in Chapter 10.

3) *Do obtain and document valid informed consents and informed refusals* (see Chapter 8).

4) *Do not use abbreviations in the records that are not universally used.* Do use only those abbreviations which would be understood by any dentist. In the case of an expert's review of the records, if the abbreviations are not understood correctly, the expert may interpret wrongly. Also, ethically, under the concept of non-malfeasance, another dentist may misinterpret your abbreviation and subsequently and inadvertently cause harm by his or her reliance on your abbreviations.

5) *Do medical consultations and document them when necessary.* It is very easy to believe you have a great understanding of the patient's complicated medical history and you are only doing a small, non-invasive procedure, and that a medical consult is not needed until the patient has an unexpected adverse reaction in your office.

6) *Do ask patients for any changes in their medical history at every appointment or as necessary.* There are many changes that may occur to a patient between appointments that the patients think are unimportant to dentistry but in reality have a great impact (True Case 16).

7) *Do inform the patient and document it when things go wrong.* The sooner the patient is told and understands the complication or bad result, the sooner the statute of limitations start tolling. Of course, it is best to correct the situation if possible.

8) *Do not practice beyond your ability.* Knowing your limitations is one of the best ways to prevent a lawsuit. If you are attempting a newer procedure, be sure to have been properly trained and have informed the patient that the procedure is new, such that a valid informed consent occurred.

9) *Do not practice beyond the scope of dentistry as defined in your state.* Many states do not allow Botox, collagen injections, rhinoplasties, or other such procedures to be done by dentists. Writing a prescription for an employee who you think only has a cold and who delays treatment, only to end up in the hospital with a more serious condition due to detrimentally relying on your advice and prescription, may cause a court to find you are practicing medicine without a license. Additionally, the removal of all amalgam restorations from a patient to treat alleged allergies without a medical consultation supporting such treatment may also cause a court to find you are practicing medicine without a license.

10) *Do maintain proper medical emergency protocols and periodic employee training.* This is a necessity on all levels: ethical, legal, risk management, and practice management.

11) *Do refer patients to the proper practitioner when necessary.* Ethically, beneficence, the patient's well-being, should always be at the forefront of your patient care. The standard of care requires you to properly refer the patient.

12) *Do not allow patients to dictate what treatment should be done.* Although patient autonomy is important, the ethical cornerstone of nonmaleficence also comes into consideration such that the dentist may not participate in the patient's self-injury. In other words, the dentist must not perform treatment that is not in the patient's best interests.

13) *Do not abandon the patient.* Dentists, who have not only an ethical duty but also a duty to fulfill the standard of care, must be available or arrange for after-hours emergency care for their patients. Do not allow the staff to deflect all patient inquiries when they ask to speak to the doctor. Finish all treatment in a timely manner.

14) *Do be available or make arrangements for patient care 24 hours a day, 7 days a week.* A dentist's not being available is one of the top reasons lawsuits are initiated.

15) *Do not discriminate or be biased.* Be professional, fair, and just to all.

16) *Do not accept litigious people as patients.* It is difficult to see the unspoken intent of a patient intending to sue regardless of the treatment rendered. Watch out for "patient setups" such as: "You're the doctor, whatever you think is best" or "Do you guarantee your work?"

17) *Do not return a fee without a Release of Liability (also called a Release of All Claims).* The return of a fee without such a signed document may be used to show guilt or the dentist's consent that treatment was wrong. Include an anti-defamation clause when terminating the doctor-patient relationship.

18) *Do not sue a patient to recover a fee unless you have reviewed the treatment rendered and the chart and know that they will be able to survive the scrutiny of a malpractice claim by the patient.* It is highly advisable to pursue other avenues of collection prior to any lawsuit, including those in small claims court, to collect a fee. Phone calls, internal office letters, and a collection agency familiar with health care collections may be a better route to collect fees. Prior to any collection effort, always talk only to the patient (due to the Health Insurance Portability and Accountability Act [HIPAA]) or guardian (if the patient is under 18) and be understanding of the patient's situation. Endodontic and prosthodontic treatments are easy targets for an unhappy patient's attorney.

19) *Do not assign employees illegal job duties.* Be fully aware of your state's allowed auxiliary job duties. For each employee who has any type of licensure, update yearly as needed to make sure he or she is still registered or licensed.

20) *Do listen to what is being said by your staff.* There are many situations that occur in the dental office of which the dentist is not aware due to the fact that he or she is normally busy treating patients. The staff may create an unnecessary problem not only by what is said but also by their attitude toward a patient. Additionally, patients notice disgruntled employees or if intra-office bickering is allowed to interfere with patient care and staff interaction.

21) *Do not have staff block patients' phone calls.* Patients often feel they are justified and understood better if only they could speak to the doctor. Most times the patient only needs to express his or her concerns. In this way a small problem can be kept from becoming a major one.

22) *Do check out references of new employees.* Always try to put trust in a newly hired employee to substantiate that your decision to hire the person was a good decision (see Chapters 15 and 24).

23) *Do keep a sample of employees' signatures,* written initials and office software passwords. When a lawsuit strikes, there will be questions regarding who made which entries in the chart. Years may pass by and employees come and go. You may have only an undecipherable scribbled initialling to which to refer or have a need for an audit trial of the patient or office records.

24) *Do have all employees trained per OSHA, HIPAA, infection control, blood-borne pathogens, and Heptevax-vaccinated regulations.* It's the law.

25) *Do document employee training and necessary periodic meetings.* When having an office meeting, always discuss topics as required by law and keep a log or sign-in sheet to verify that employee training is ongoing.

26) *Do maintain adequate malpractice insurance that will cover any new treatment you are providing.* With the advance of newer procedures and the expanded continuing education courses available, always contact your insurance company as to how these new treatment modalities (e.g., implants or Botox) will affect your malpractice insurance.

27) *Do keep all the billing proper.* Use the correct treatment codes and do not "expand" or "upgrade" to a better paying code. This type of misrepresentation is fraudulent billing. If the insurance-authorized treatment is different from that which you and the patient believe is proper, then write an appeal explaining the situation rather than simply billing wrongly.

28) *Do not overbill or double-bill the patient's dental insurance company.* Do not accept the dental insurance payment as full payment when it is meant to be a percentage of the fee and forgive the patient's portion of payment. When the patient portion or percentage of the bill is forgiven when the insurance only pays a percentage of the total bill, then the true total billing is the amount the insurance paid. Hence the insurance paid 100% of the bill when it should have paid only a percentage of the bill. This type of fraudulent billing is not covered under your malpractice insurance.

29) *Do review patient charts daily.* Daily or at least weekly, the dentist should skim through the charts of the previous day or days to make sure entries are correct, proper follow-through by the staff is occurring (patient has a next visit appointment or has been placed in a notebook to be have follow-up phone call), and to have the opportunity to make a "late entry," if necessary, when recollection is clearest.

30) *Do call patients the night after surgery, root canal, or an extensive treatment or problem.* By doing so, the dentist will be able to pick up on any post-treatment problem such as unforeseen pain, bleeding, or swelling. Also, it is a great practice enhancement since patients appreciate the concern shown in a follow-up call.

31) *Do periodically review patient bills and insurance forms the staff has been submitting.* There have been cases against dentists for fraudulent billing by a partner or staff member, while the dentist had no idea that it had occurred. Nevertheless, you will be held responsible via vicarious liability/respondeat superior.

32) *Do check expiration dates on all supplies.* If an employee is given this job duty, be sure to check up on his or her progress once in a while to make sure emergency drugs, anesthetics, and other such items are safe.

33) *Do complete exams before extensive treatment.* Many patients are new to a practice due to an emergency such as pain, swelling, or a fractured tooth or denture. Inevitably, after the

emergency is treated successfully, the new patient will seek treatment for other dental concerns. Rather than treating each patient concern or emergency as it arises, a complete exam and treatment plan should take place to prevent improper treatment outcomes (radiographs, PSR-periodontal screening, cancer screening, temporomandibular joint [TMJ] screening).

34) *Do keep treatment plans prioritized: pain, infection, function, aesthetics.* Many treatment plans may become multifaceted and require treatment to take place over numerous months or even years. To keep the patient and yourself on track with a proposed treatment plan that changes due to the lapse in time to complete, break down the treatment so the patient can easily understand that priorities will be patient-centered and that treatment will be provided first for pain, then infection, function, and aesthetics.

35) *Do have the patient understand his or her financial responsibilities before treatment is rendered.* As emphasized under informed consent, cost is often a determining factor in a patient's consent to the proposed treatment (patient financing issues are discussed in Chapter 21).

36) *Do not promise or guarantee treatment outcomes.* To guarantee treatment outcomes is against the standard of care. Watch out for the "setups" (discussed in Chapter 12).

37) *Do not make statements that may be used against you.* Statements against your interest that are made at the time of an event or incident may be used against you in a court of law (Res Gestae Exception to Hearsay). The statements made by employees may also be used against you. So be very careful that you or your employees do not blurt out, "Oh no," "Oops," or any other exclamation that may alarm the patient and be used against you in a court of law depending on your jurisdiction. Remain professional and calm when situations arise that may be less than ideal.

38) *Be aware of your state's agency laws.* This will affect how you are responsible for your associate dentists and when covering a colleague's practice while he or she is away or unable to work due to sickness or injury.

Collections

Many lawsuits have started due to the pursuit of collection of a balance the patient owes. Prior to seeking collection be sure to review the chart and make sure all treatment was well above the standard of care. Also evaluate if the amount sought is worth the time spent on seeking payment. One of the best ways is to set up a system for collection of fees that are not made in a timely manner. Besides the normal billing cycle of the office, a simple phone call may resolve the issue. Any contact or message/letter sent should be noted on a separate sheet of paper from the patient treatment chart because it is not patient care related. If phone contact has been made or a message left, be sure to follow up at a certain date. Failure to make contact again on that date gives a message that payment is not that important to the office and affects the office credibility in the pursuit of collection. Patients also have unforeseen situations such as a lost job, lost insurance coverage, sickness, etc., that might have affected their payments. Be understanding of such situations and work with the patient to resolve the payment problem. Upon full payment, a forgiveness of any accrued interest or a courtesy percentage discount may help show you being helpful and understanding of the situation. Sometimes, it is only that the patient moved and was not aware of the balance due because of a change of address.

Here are some suggestions for the collection process:

1) Internal letter on letterhead requesting payment. When signing the letter be sure to write "If there are any problems we should be aware of, please call the office." This is then followed-up two weeks later with a phone call.
2) A delinquency form (available on the Internet) should be sent and again followed-up with a phone call two weeks later.
3) Seek outside collection agency if deemed necessary.

If You Are Sued

Approximately one in seven dentists will be sued during his or her professional career. That statistic takes into consideration the fact that some dentists may be sued several times and others never as seen in True Case 35. Also, many people sue for reasons other than having been damaged, for example, the patient needs money, dislikes the staff and/or the dentist, doesn't want to pay the bill, or has a relative who is an attorney. Also, some unethical attorneys may pursue cases for the need to keep busy or to pay rent. Patients may be angry or dislike the dentist for a variety of reasons: the dentist makes too much money, or the patient is in pain and the dentist seems unsympathetic. It is how you handle these types of patients and what you do after things do not work out as planned that makes a big difference in whether or not the patient seeks legal advice.

True Case 35: (True Case 6 revisited): Dentist leaves state
A state dental board requested a review of several malpractice cases against the same dentist. It was revealed that there were seven cases for review with more pending against this dentist, and the state board wanted to revoke his license. During the process of review and eventual revocation, the dentist relinquished his license to the state board only after he applied for and received a license in another state. Hence, some dentists account for more than that one in seven.

Nevertheless, you need to know what to do in case you find yourself as a defendant in a lawsuit. First, if you have employed proper risk management techniques and treatment protocols, you should reassure yourself that being named in the lawsuit does not mean you did anything wrong. It will be very stressful to the point that you may experience Medical Malpractice Syndrome as discussed in Chapter 1. As mentioned before, some patients are just litigious people who cannot be foreseen. Being sued affects you emotionally in that you start to question yourself and begin doubting your treatment. You will be hesitant to provide that treatment again for awhile. Do not panic; these are normal reactions or feelings. Do not call the patient or the patient's attorney. Call your malpractice insurance company immediately. A claims advisor will be most helpful in guiding you through the situation. First remove the chart from general circulation within your office. Review the chart carefully, acting as a "devil's advocate" and questioning your chart for completeness and integrity. On a separate sheet of paper to be kept apart from the file, write down to the best of your recollection what happened. Do not talk to any colleagues regarding the case. Only talk to staff on an as-needed basis. Above all, do not write in the chart or make any changes to the chart like the dentist in True Case 36.

True Case 36: (True Case 2 revisited): Changing the chart

After being an expert witness many times, you can usually get a feeling on how the jury is accepting your testimony, in other words, whether the jury is accepting the expert's testimony as the truth. The credibility of the expert witness's testimony is paramount in establishing a solid defense. In this example, after successfully making a solid defense for the dentist, the plaintiff's attorney started to cross-examine. The defense failed to show substandard care. Then the expert was asked to read what was written at the top of page three of the patient's chart. After reading what was written, the plaintiff's attorney asked to read what was above that which was just read. The expert said his copy had nothing written above. The plaintiff's attorney proceeded to produce a copy of the patient's chart that had been altered by the dentist after copies were made. Rather than win the case easily, not only did the dentist lose the case, but the jury came back with damages far exceeding that which was originally sought. Therefore, do not make changes to the chart!

Make complete copies of the chart, including radiographs (if digital, make sure the image is clear as possible), the attorney's letter, and any other correspondence. Do not give the originals to anyone, including your attorney. Give the originals only on a court-ordered, subpoenaed request. Attorney's offices are just like any other office in which things fall out of folders and get lost. With today's digital imaging and computerized records, the chance of lost records is lessened, but things can still be accidentally miss-entered or even deleted. Be sure to check your malpractice insurance if there is a settlement clause whereby the insurance company may settle your case against your approval, or where you may be responsible for any amount above the insurance-approved settlement amount if the successful claim is higher. If the claim is significant and may be beyond or close to your coverage limits, retain a personal attorney to protect you personally.

During any examinations before trial (depositions, arbitrations, settlement hearings) always dress professionally. Answer questions only if you are absolutely positive of the answer. Do not guess the answer or try to impress the attorney, judge, or jury. If you do not know the answer or do not understand the question, simply say so. If necessary, ask to hear the question again or to have it rephrased. Do not lie or try to outwit the attorney. He or she has been trained to ask leading questions that may lead you down the wrong path, which you will not realize until it is too late. There are also those questions in which the attorney rephrases your previous answer in a following question; such as, "Isn't it true that ___," "You are aware that___," or "You said that____," which you need to be aware that it sounding similar to what you said but is phrased a little differently. Always be sincere in your answers and polite. Do not show anger or contempt.

There is no way anyone can predict the outcome of a lawsuit due to the many players and facets involved: dentist, patient, dentist's attorney, patient's attorney, expert witnesses, judge, and jury. Most dental cases are settled before trial, as the costs of a trial are high and the damages, relatively speaking, are small.

To settle or not to settle is the question often asked. The following question should help guide that decision:

1) Are you in the right and defensible?
2) Would you make a good witness?
3) Is there a deductible applied by your malpractice insurance?
4) Is there a "consent to settle" clause in malpractice insurance?

5) What are the consequences of settling the claim such as reporting to NPDB and/or your state's professional discipline agency?
6) Are you able to settle the claim by paying it personally?

Practice Enhancement Through Risk Management

Both practice enhancement and risk management discussions have a basis in good patient communications. Through risk management, dentists attempt to prevent lawsuits by informing patients (and receiving their consent) through proper communication. In practice enhancement, dentists attempt to have patients accept a treatment plan of optimum dental care through communication [6]. Risk management began as a tool to strengthen a dentist defendant's defense in a malpractice lawsuit. It is also builds your dental practice when applied properly.

The 2005 ADA survey of 15 dental malpractice insurance companies uncovered the top three dentist–patient communication problems:

1) Critical comments of the insured's work made to a patient by another dentist.
2) Professional liability claims filed in retaliation for billing or collection problems.
3) Lack of or poor communication between a primary dentist and a specialist [7].

The total inclusion of the patient in the decision-making discussion truly enhances the practice and manages malpractice risks. Risk management actually begins prior to the patient entering the dental office. Communication with the patient begins in the external marketing/advertising of the practice and the image or perception of the dental office. Prospective patients have an impression of the office through the direct discussion/referral from another patient, external advertising, Internet websites, and dental insurance information/provider lists. Prospective patients' impressions are also affected by the internal marketing of the practice through the manner in which the first phone call is handled, office décor, office cleanliness, and proper scheduling. All these things make an impression on the prospective patient before the first entry into any chart is ever made. That impression adds to or takes away from the trust that should develop in a positive doctor–patient relationship. The more the trust the patient has in the dentist and the office, the less chance of a falsely accused malpractice lawsuit and the patient questioning whether the dentist's treatment is or was right. Involve the whole dental team in risk management. Staff members should be encouraged to inform you of potential risk exposure by promoting a blame-free environment such that the staff feels comfortable to point out any problems.

Once the patient has filled out all the proper initial visit forms, the dentist and the entire dental staff must take part in developing a trusting doctor–patient relationship. Before the dentist ever meets the patient, there have been at least three patient contacts made that have already influenced the patient's attitude toward the dentist and his or her office:

1) How the phone is answered.
2) How the patient is welcomed to the office and requested to fill required forms.
3) How the assistant or hygienist greet and treat the patient.

The dental staff is very much a part of the risk management effort. Communication is necessary not only between the patient and the office but also between the staff and the dentist as seen in True Case 37. Without proper intra-office communication, patient care may not be optimum.

True Case 37: Who knows what is going on?

The patient showed up on time for her appointment for the crown preparation of a molar. The patient was in need of several crowns, including #18 and #19. The schedule only noted that the appointment was for a crown on the lower left. The dentist anaesthetized the lower left. Knowing the patient wanted to have only one crown due to the expenses and that only one of the two teeth was approved by the insurance company because of yearly maximum limits, he proceeded to prepare the worst of the two needed crowns on the lower left, #18. During the appointment, the assistant noticed in the chart that tooth #19 was actually the tooth approved by the insurance company. The dentist immediately informed the patient of the mis-communication and stated that if it was okay with the patient, he would also do the tooth that was approved by the insurance company since it was already numb. The patient agreed but questioned if she would have to pay for the other tooth already started but not covered by insurance. The dentist, ethically and legally accepting the fact that he had prepared the wrong tooth, explained to the patient that #18 was the worse of the two teeth and that he was sorry for the mix up. He then informed her that there would be no charge, but if at all possible, she should cover the lab fee. The patient, knowing that the tooth did need the crown, agreed to cover the lab fee, and was thankful to the dentist for being honest about it.

Further discussion on the development of the dental team and their influence on the doctor–patient relationship may be found in Chapter 22 and in "Leadership and Communication in Dentistry."

The Examination

The initial exam in any situation other than emergencies should include, but should not be limited to, a complete examination, a full medical–dental history (as discussed in Chapter 6), measurement of blood pressure and pulse, periodontal charting or a periodontal screening report (PSR), cancer screening, TMJ screening, a full set of radiographs, and a caries/restorative examination. The examination may entail more diagnostics (such as more intraoral photographs, endodontic testing, scans/cone beam images), depending on the treatment needs of the patient. On examination, any diagnostic procedures performed and the results therefrom must be recorded, a treatment plan must be developed, the patient must be informed, and the treatment or refusal of treatment must be recorded, or the patient should be referred to the proper professional.

It is strongly advised to perform a complete periodontal charting on any patient more than 25 years old or on those younger if indicated via radiographic or visual examination. If the radiographic and visual examination does not reveal a need for complete periodontal charting on patients under 25, then a PSR as promoted by the ADA and the American Academy of Periodontists may be sufficient. It is an easy and quick way to screen for periodontitis. Simply "walk" the periodontal probe around each tooth and spot check areas of concern as indicated on the radiographs or as visually observed. Then divide the mouth into six parts (sextants) and record the deepest pocket in each section. A code of 0–4 is then given to each section. A section with a code of 0 (all probings ≤3 millimeters, no bleeding, no calculus, and no defects) is healthy and only requires routine preventive care. A section with a code of 1 (all probings ≤3 millimeters, bleeding present, no calculus, and no defects) requires subgingival plague removal. A section with a code of 2 (all probings ≤3 millimeters and supra- and subgingival calculus present) requires subgingival calculus removal. A section with a code of 3 (probing >3 millimeters and <5 millimeters and supra- and subgingival calculus present) requires full mouth charting and scaling. A section with a code of 4 (probings >5 millimeters, supra- and subgingival calculus present, and osseous defects) requires full mouth charting, scaling, and root planning, as well as referral to a periodontal specialist or further periodontal treatment after re-evaluation [8]. Oral hygiene instruction should always be given to a patient, including the proper cleaning under bridges, around implants, and proper cleansing of removable appliances.

Patients older than 25 years should also receive a cancer screening (younger if the patient is a smoker or in another high-risk group), and a TMJ screening if temporomandibular dysfunction (TMD) was present prior to any treatment rendered (this prevents a claim of causing iatrogenic TMD).

Having good diagnostic skills is an important step in risk management but also in practice enhancement, because if you do not diagnose it, you will not treat it. As a result of skilled diagnostic time with the patient, the practice will have improved production and, subsequently, profit. Even with superior diagnostics, the most important factor in preventing a lawsuit may be left out: trust. The dentist must gain the patient's trust to truly allow practice enhancement through risk management to take place. To gain the patient's trust, the dentist must strive to include the patient in all treatment discussion to the level of actually having the patient "co-diagnose" his or her dental needs.

If the digital images (both radiographs and intraoral photos) are the size of the monitor screen, it is relatively easy to show and involve the patient. By listening to the patient about what is perceived as his or her dental needs and wants, the dentist is able to bring the patient into the treatment plan discussion. Once you understand the patient's concerns, desires, and expectations, you can turn his or her needs into wants through an educational discussion, thereby raising the patient's "dental IQ" one notch. It is advised to empathize and to understand the patient's life from the patient's perspective. He or she has numerous other responsibilities and obligations that may impact the decision-making process. Through this discussion, the dentist is developing a trusting doctor–patient relationship that decreases the chances of a lawsuit, since the patient is trusting and the avenues of communication are open in case of an unexpected problem.

Treatment plans may be confusing to a patient with limited dental knowledge. To help clarify the proposed treatment and its sequence, it is best to prioritize the treatment in a way the patient can understand it. The treatment plan should be prioritized, as previously discussed, into four categories: pain, infection, function, and aesthetics. Of course, there are times when these categories intermingle and must be considered equally at the time of treatment [9]. More time should be spent discussing the results of the proposed treatment rather than how the treatment will be done or how well the dentist can do it. Patients perceive dental care, except when in pain, as a discretionary expense; they view it with respect to what value the proposed treatment will have in their lives. Raising the value of treatment to the patient by raising his or her understanding (dental IQ), the patient's needs turn into wants. What has developed is an enhancement to the practice when patients understand the need and value of the proposed treatment, and a fulfillment of risk management for the practice when the patient has developed a full trust in an understanding, knowledgeable, and caring dentist. Normally, people do not sue people they trust.

Beware of the patient setups and doctor/staff "oops" and "oh-no"s. Statements/utterances against your self-interest that are made at the time of injury or occurrence may be used against you. Dentist set ups include statements such as:

"I can save that tooth."
"I can give you a perfect smile."
"When I'm done, your teeth will be perfectly straight."
"It will be just like your own teeth again."
"This extraction will be easy."

Patient set ups include statements such as:

"Just do the best you can. I trust you."
"You don't have to tell me about the procedure, I've had it done before."
"Do whatever you think is best."
"My last dentist didn't know what he was doing. I've heard you're the best."
"You did such a great job on my husband's teeth. I want the same."

Patients with dental emergencies often need immediate attention. Often these types of appointments are rushed. When fitting an emergency patient into a tight schedule, some of the usual patient evaluations may inadvertently be sidestepped. When the emergency patient comes in, be sure to follow proper patient medical history evaluation, including taking blood pressure. Full documentation of emergency treatment is a must. The "SOAP" rule is the best example of how to organize the emergency:

S: Subjective comment of the patient. It is the patient's chief complaint.
O: Objective evaluation. These are your diagnostic tools and their findings used to evaluate the patient's chief complaint.
A: Assessment, analysis, diagnosis. This is the differential diagnosis of the patient's complaint.
P: Plan the treatment. This is the treatment plan with alternatives rendering a successful treatment of the patient's complaint and needs.

There are also the medical emergencies that may erupt unexpectedly. Legally and ethically, you need to be prepared and up-to-date with emergency training and protocols, equipment, and medications. You also are expected to have your staff properly trained in emergency situations that might occur. An office meeting once or twice a year to reinforce emergency situation responsibilities and training/drills helps to keep everyone up-to-date and attentive to potential emergencies.

The scheduling of the patient is another key to practice enhancement through risk management. Enough time must be given to properly develop a trusting doctor–patient relationship. Some patients require more time than others. When insufficient time is allotted, the patient perceives the dentist as rushed and uncaring. Therefore, it is important to properly schedule sufficient time to allow the patient to ask any questions and feel he or she has the dentist's full focus during the dental visit. Even long-term patients may find their trust in the dentist slipping if the dentist begins to take the patient's trust for granted or does not focus entirely on the patient. Therefore, it is always good to remember that there is a mutual investment in the doctor–patient relationship that must always be protected.

Once the patient leaves the office, the practice enhancement through risk management continues. After any traumatic treatment such as endodontic therapy, periodontal surgery, or extractions, making a follow-up call that evening or the next day promotes the quality of care, keeps you aware of any patient concerns, and allows you to prevent those unexpected problems that unnecessarily complicate the doctor–patient relationship. It is always better for the dentist to head off a situation rather than to wait for the patient to question a situation that would weaken the previously built trust.

Another important step in risk prevention is to review the charts from the previous day or days before they are filed away, to be aware of any small problems. There are three things to look for:

1) Did the patient make a next appointment or was the patient placed on the proper maintenance recall?
2) If the patient did not make an appointment, was the patient placed on a "to be called" list, or in some kind of notebook that lists those patients who need to be called for a follow-up appointment?
3) Are the chart notes accurate and complete?

If any problem is found with the above, easy and fast correction may be made prior to a small situation developing into a massive miscommunication. It is also an excellent way to make any notes that were inadvertently missed. If you do, do not change the chart. Date a new entry, mark it as a "late entry," make your notation, and sign it. Your best chance to make the addition properly is when your recollection is clearest. If the change is substantial, then the patient must be informed of the change at the next visit (if reasonably soon), must be called to discuss the change, or should come in to have his or her understanding clarified and the chart entry rectified. Making a late entry is a rare occurrence, but the accuracy and truthfulness of the chart is paramount.

Therefore, five major practice enhancements exist from using good risk management techniques:

1) Improve the quality of practice.
2) Improve practice production.
3) Improve practice profits.
4) Decrease the practitioner's stress.
5) Decrease the costs to defend malpractice lawsuits.

By using simple, time-effective risk management techniques, the dentist will also find an increase in treatment plan acceptance by trusting patients through proper communication and co-diagnosis. Through the proper patient communication by the doctor and the staff, a great doctor–patient relationship will develop, such that risk management is easily accomplished and the threat of a lawsuit is greatly lessened.

References

1 ADA Council on Members Insurance and Retirement Programs, *1999–2003 Insurance Company Survey*, 2003, p. 5.
2 Ibid., p. 6.
3 Ibid., p. 4.
4 Joseph Graskemper, "A New Perspective on Dental Malpractice," *Journal of the American Dental Association*, Vol. 133 (June 2002), p. 752.
5 Ibid., p. 753.
6 Ibid.
7 ADA Council on Members Insurance and Retirement Programs, *1999–2003 Insurance Company Survey*, 2003, p. 10.
8 Graskemper, "A New Perspective on Dental Malpractice," p. 755.
9 Ibid.

15

Employees and Associates

A dentist has risk exposure if he or she has employees or associates. Although a full discussion on labor/employment law is beyond the scope of this book, the dentist should be made aware of the basics. The employer/dentist carries responsibility for his or her employees under the doctrine of respondeat superior, which is applied to the dentist under vicarious liability law (see the definitions in Chapter 3). It is that part of vicarious liability law that applies to the employer–employee relationships. Under respondeat superior, the employer:

1) Selects the employee to act.
2) Controls employee activities.
3) Benefits from employee activities.

Hence, since the employer benefits from the employee's activities, the employer assumes the risk of the employee's activities.

Associates may be found to be not only as employees but rather independent contractors. Recently, the Internal Revenue Service (IRS) changed the criteria regarding the associate's status as to whether the associate would be considered an employee or an independent contractor. The new IRS test is wider in scope to include more into the independent contractor status. However, naming an associate an independent contractor and fulfilling any IRS criteria to be an independent contractor does not totally shield the owner dentist from liability due to various agency laws The IRS test is an 11-part assessment divided into three categories:

1) Behavior control
2) Financial control
3) Type of relationship [1].

Employee/independent contractor status is covered in more detail in Chapter 19.

Referring to another health care practitioner or specialist also has risks attached. There is normally no liability when referring to a specialist unless:

1) The referring dentist knew or should have known the specialist is impaired or incompetent.
2) The referring dentist materially benefited from the referral.
3) The referring dentist directed or took part in the treatment provided by the specialist.

With the growth of multispecialty practices, husband/wife/related family practices, and itinerant specialists working out of general dentist's offices, the owner dentist must understand the risks and benefits of referring to intra-office associates or specialists. Such multidoctor offices are beneficial to both doctors and patients. Having multiple doctors working together in one office

Professional Responsibility in Dentistry: A Practical Guide to Law and Ethics, Second Edition. Joseph P. Graskemper.
© 2023 John Wiley & Sons, Inc. Published 2023 by John Wiley & Sons, Inc.

lowers overhead and allows multiple specialists to work together on one patient during the same visit. Having one office where multiple specialists are available is extremely convenient to the patient. However, due to the mutual benefit arrangement of intra-office referral, the doctors carry mutual risks and may be found liable for each other (see Chapter 25).

Hiring and Firing

Hiring and firing also needs to be discussed. Hiring always seems to be a fun and exciting time, with both the employer and the employee looking forward to a positive relationship. Check references and ask yourself if this applicant is the best applicant for the practice. Do not discriminate based on age, sex, race, sexual orientation, or religion. Hence it is best not to ask questions regarding these areas. There should be a well-documented description of the job duties the newly hired employee is expected to fulfill. There should also be a clear and complete office policy manual and employee handbook in place prior to hiring an employee, to prevent any misunderstandings. It should also inform the new employee of all expectations and work rules affecting his or her job, including grounds by which they may be fired. Firing has never been found to be a happy experience by either party and is most likely to lead to problems. From the date of hire, always document all employee discussions regarding employment and job performance. When an employee is not performing his or her job duties satisfactorily, bring such deficiencies to his or her attention immediately. If a written warning is used, both the employer and the employee should sign it to prevent miscommunication, and a copy of it should be given to the employee. Normally, a three-warning system regarding the same problem is sufficient (keep in mind the baseball rule of "three strikes and you're out"). The first warning is made orally. The second is made with a standard written form (found online or any good office supply store). The third warning is also written and a decision must be made regarding termination. Always inform the employee, orally or in writing, of how to remedy the situation. It is best to try to work with a known employee to remedy a situation rather than to hire a new employee. Nevertheless, continued poor performance or not showing up for work, as shown in True Case 38, are grounds for termination. Firing should not be emotional. It should be based on fact. You should have a witness at the time of firing to extinguish any miscommunication or misunderstanding. Even with proper documentation, a disgruntled employee may file for unemployment due to financial or emotional motives to get even with the employer.

True Case 38: Extra-long vacation

An employee informed the dentist that she was going on vacation for one week. She was the only dental assistant for this dentist, as it was a small office. She had been employed by the dentist for over two years, and it was a trip that she had been planning a long time. They both marked the office calendar so all team members were aware of her week-long absence. On the day when she was due back, the dentist received a phone call that she would be away one more day. The dentist, although a little upset, approved her request to take one more day of vacation. When the next day came and the dental assistant did not show up for work, he called but could not reach her. The second day past the original due date, again no contact was possible

---

(Continued)

True Case 38 (Continued)

with the employee. The dentist assumed she quit and hired another person. Three days after she was due back, she showed up for work. On being fired, she filed for unemployment benefits. The dentist appealed the decision to grant her benefits due to her unexcused absence of three days after she was due to return to work. At the hearing with an administrative law judge, the assistant and her mother showed the judge that her airline ticket and her calendar were marked properly regarding to the extra days off, and she denied calling to ask for extra days off. Even with letters from other staff members that the employee had made the phone call and was due back sooner, the judge granted unemployment benefits to the employee. It was later found that the employee changed her flight to stay longer on vacation.

Unemployment

When an employee files for unemployment after being fired, you will receive a form stating that the employee filed unemployment against you and the reason why you should be responsible for it. If your state allows an "at will" contract for employment, be sure to state that in the Office Policy Manual (as discussed in Chapter 10, in "Leadership and Communication in Dentistry"). If you want to contest the filing you must give a reason why. The reason for firing is normally insubordination or misconduct and the particulars that relate to the firing. When you contest the filing, the case will normally go to an Administrative Judge who normally follows rules and regulation of the National Labor Relations Board and jurisdictional laws that apply. Even if the employee worked only a day in a working interview like the employee in True Case 39, you could be held liable for unemployment. In such cases, it should be pro-rated with previous employers.

True Case 39: Just eight hours count

The dentist hired an applicant for a dental assistant position. It was agreed that there would be a 90 day try-out period to make sure both were happy working together. The dentist was only open for the mornings on the first two days of the try-out period. The new hiree was a nightmare and after the second half day she was let go to find another office. The following week the dentist received notice that she filed for unemployment. He appealed the decision based on the fact that she was only trying out for the position and not fully hired until the try-out period ended. The Administrative Judge ruled that even if she only worked 10 minutes, she is able to claim unemployment benefits. It was stated that the time spent is not the determining fact. If she was paid for the time spent for the try-out period, then she has the benefit of unemployment, although it would be pro-rated with previous employers.

Employee activities that are allowed include, but not limited to, concerted union forming activities, use of social media among themselves against the employer, and disparaging and abusive words toward the employer among themselves. You cannot stop employees from talking to each other. In other words, almost anything the employee says or does will more likely than not be allowed, except physical threats and acts (assault and battery).

Staff Snafus/Problems

Not having a written Office Policy Manual causes a lot of misunderstandings within the office. Without it, there is no guidance as to what is expected from the staff, their interactions among themselves and with patients, and what is expected from the employer. Without such guidance the cohesive team that makes a practice very successful will not be able to meet their potential.

When an employee begins the downward slope of unacceptable behavior such as continual lateness, gossiping, or just plain out nasty, they will be an anchor to the practice's potential. Although attempts to work with the employee are failing, the delay in firing may cause more damage than anticipated. A bad hire or a negative change in an employee may necessitate he or she be given the opportunity to find another office by terminating their employment.

Giving too many benefits or starting the wage at hiring too high, makes it very hard to have the employee grow into the practice culture. Many times, it is viewed by fellow employees that a certain employee is given too much power (such as access to your checkbook) or has special attention (such as only giving special days off to only one employee). This will cause resentment among the other employees again hampering the success of the practice. Giving too much control or power to 1 employee can cause a lot of damage to you, the employer, and your practice as seen in True Case 40.

True Case 40: Embezzlement

The dentist had extreme trust in his receptionist giving her access to his banking information to assist him in managing the practice. After a seven-year period, the dentist started to notice that although he was very busy he had to take loans out to cover the practice expenses. He took out a second mortgage on his house to cover credit card debt and discontinued timely payments into his retirement fund. When he went to the bank for a personal loan, they informed him of the loans he already had. An audit showed forged signatures for loans and an investigation showing those funds were spent on drugs. The total amount of the embezzlement was $1,600,000.00!

There is more than money that is of high value within a dental practice. The patient information, such as, but not limited to, names, credit card information, social security numbers, email addresses, and insurance information. There are signs that may raise a question of embezzlement by certain employee activities. Be aware of an employee that wants to have full control over the processing of insurance forms or accepting patient payments, evades discussion regarding patient finances, shifts blame to co-workers and may possibly become volatile or dramatic when challenged.

To protect yourself as best you can, educate yourself on the workings of your software, check the daysheet at the end of each day or first thing in the following morning, be more visible up front and not hide in your office, and give no one access to your banking information.

Embezzlement can also occur by fraud in billing insurance companies for services. Some examples of fraud are:

1) Billing for services not rendered.
2) Waiving of deductible and/or patient portion (co-payment).
3) Misrepresentation of treatment dates.
4) Up-coding of services (all extractions be surgical).

Harassment

Of course, sexual harassment, as in any business, is not allowed in a dental practice. Sexual harassment claims are not covered by your malpractice insurance. Do not date patients or employees. There is also an ethical responsibility in which the dentist should not become involved in a patient/employee relationship where one of the persons may feel coerced or threatened into the relationship.

There are many types of harassment that can become actionable by the patient or the employee:

Verbal – most common.
Inappropriate communication.
Inappropriate behavior.
Hostile work environment.
Cyber/Social media communication.
Sexual – most actionable and hardest to defend.

Sexual harassment is not covered by your malpractice insurance. There is insurance to cover unintended harassment of patients and/or employees. The best way to prevent such an allegation is to be very careful of any personal relationship with patients and/or employees. Be aware that harassment is viewed from the person being allegedly harassed as seen in True Case 41(it's not always who you would think). So be very careful that the simple hug or pat on the back is not taken wrongly.

True Case 41: Looks too good

In Nelson v. Knight, Dr. Knight won a case involving the firing of a dental assistant because she was too attractive. She worked for Dr. Knight for over 10 years. He stated to her that her "clothing was too tight, revealing and distracting," that she was "a big threat to his marriage," "she did nothing wrong or inappropriate," and "feared he would try to have an affair with her down the road." [2]

   You just never know or expect how the court will rule.

References

1 Peter Sfikas, "IRS' New Test," *Dental Practice Report* (May 2007), p. 54.
2 Melissa Nelson, Appellant, v. James H. Knight DDS, P.C., and James Knight, "Appellees, Supreme Court of Iowa," No. 11–1857, decided: July 12, 2013.

Part III

Professionalism and Ethics

16

Professionalism

A profession is different from an occupation. Your interaction with a professional is different from interactions with nonprofessionals. A professional has certain privileges, obligations, responsibilities, and risks. A profession has been defined as "a collective of expert service providers who jointly and publicly [are] committed to always give priority to the existential needs and interests of the public they serve above their own and who, in turn, are trusted by the public to do so" [1]. In a more inclusive definition derived from the Oxford English Dictionary and various literature on professionalism, a profession is an occupation whose core element is work based on the mastery of a complex body of knowledge and skills. It is a vocation in which knowledge of some department of science or learning or the practice of an art is used in the service of others. Its members are governed by codes of ethics, and profess a commitment to competence, integrity and morality, altruism, and to the promotion of the public good within their domain. These commitments form the basis of a social contract between a profession and society, which in turn grants the profession a monopoly over the use of its knowledge base, the right to considerable autonomy in practice, and the privilege of self-regulation. Professions and their members are accountable to those served and to society. Hence, there is a social contract between the professional and the people he or she serves. Dentists have special knowledge and skills by being able to diagnose and treat illness and disease. Dentists possess special privileges to ask private questions, to prescribe medications, and to perform surgery. Dentists also have special responsibilities of self-regulation and to put the patient's welfare first. Therefore, dentistry is a profession fulfilling the definitions mentioned earlier. Hence, a professional dentist will not capitalize on the vulnerability of patients in an attempt to maximize his or her own interests and will live up to the trust that the public and every patient places in him or her and in dentistry as a whole. The public trust must be sustained if the profession will continue under a social contract.

Professional Obligations

There are nine categories of professional obligation:

1) The chief client: This is the person or set of persons whose well-being the profession and its members are chiefly committed to serving; from the patient currently being treated by the dentist or the public as a whole by the entire dental community.
2) The ideal relationship between dentist and patient: The relationship should bring certain values to the client, values that cannot be achieved for the client without the expertise of the professional. This can be achieved by involving the patient in a co-diagnosing relationship.

Professional Responsibility in Dentistry: A Practical Guide to Law and Ethics, Second Edition. Joseph P. Graskemper.
© 2023 John Wiley & Sons, Inc. Published 2023 by John Wiley & Sons, Inc.

3) The central values of the dental professional: A profession is focused only on certain aspects of the well-being of its clients from the patient's general and oral health to patient autonomy and use of resources.

4) Competence: Every professional is obligated both to acquire and to maintain the expertise needed to undertake his or her professional tasks (this can also be seen in the 10 elements of the standard of care in Chapter 13). Applying the risk/benefit of treatment to all patients in a professional and ethical manner.

5) Sacrifice and the relative priority of the patient's well-being: A profession obligates its members to accept significant sacrifices that are neither unlimited nor unqualified, such that dentists as professionals also have autonomy in their patient care decisions within the standard of care.

6) Ideal relationship between co-professionals: Professionals should work together as collaborators for the patient's well-being.

7) The relationship between dentistry and the larger community: Professionals are obliged to also collaborate with those other than patients and co-professionals, such as dental hygienists and office staff, and those outside direct patient care, who have an interest in the well-being of the patient, such as pharmacists, physicians, nurses, dental manufacturers/suppliers, and dental labs.

8) Availability of services: Professionals will attempt to serve all of society, including those with special needs and those who do not have access to adequate dental care, through charity and public dental health programs.

9) Integrity and education: A professional not only works by a set of ethical values but also lives by them [2].

These nine obligations required of dentistry in order for it to be a profession may also be condensed and presented in a set of three inquiries:

1) Who serves?
2) What kind of service is provided?
3) Who is served? [3]

A profession must ensure that its members are competent to serve the public. Dentistry has set up specific schools of dentistry and a set of benchmark tests (state boards/regional boards/residencies) to create a standard for the competency of dentists. Not anyone may become a dentist, even if tutored by another licensed dentist. Without graduating from a dental school and passing a dental board, graduate residency program, or portfolio competency, one cannot be a dentist. The profession must govern itself. Peer review, as discussed in Chapter 13, assesses colleagues through a review by their peers. A profession must be able to discipline those who have not maintained or who have breached the social contract. All state boards of dentistry have the powers directly or indirectly through another agency to reprimand, suspend, or revoke a dentist's license. Therefore, there is a responsibility for the profession to maintain controls over who will serve as a professional. Through various means of testing, peer reviews, and disciplinary actions, it is ensured that all dentists are competent to fulfill dentistry's social contract.

A profession must provide services that are objectively fulfilling a public need. There is no question as to the need for dental services. Nevertheless, how does dentistry objectively fulfill that needed service? There are many agencies, groups, schools, and associations that reach that goal through empirical sciences, research, statistic gathering, and outcome assessments. To fulfill that goal objectively, these various groups must assess different new and upcoming treatment modalities/protocols as to their effectiveness and efficiency and introduce objectively positive developments into the dental services provided. Therefore, there is a standardization of treatment protocols or a standard of care that is provided by dentists for the benefit of the public. There are also the many agencies, both public and private, which help provide dental care for those in need.

Finally, a profession's goal must be to serve the public that allows the profession to exist, without discrimination. Dentists should be altruistic in their treatment of all patients and not refuse treatment to certain patients, or limit or restrict access to needed dental care. This is not to say dentists should provide free treatment for all patients with a dental need. It is inevitable that a conflict of interest will exist: providing care for those in need and providing income to cover financial responsibilities. However, the dentist, being a professional, must acknowledge that conflict and try to minimize it. The ethical professional dentist will at times reach out and help those in need without a continual quest for income, whether it is by providing care for reduced reimbursement or providing care at no charge. Dentistry has always supported public and private endeavors to help treat those in need through public assistance programs and volunteerism.

In fulfilling the requirements of being members of a profession, dentists must exhibit professionalism. Professionalism is the conduct or qualities that a person must have to be a professional. The attributes that make up a professional are many and diverse. Some of the qualities that are normally seen in a professional are compassion, kindness, integrity, fairness, and charity (service-mindedness). Other attributes include respect for others, accountability, professional responsibility, striving for excellence, altruism, and a commitment to social justice (fairness), and a willingness to acknowledge errors. Being a professional also carries with it the weight of self-assessment. Dentists should constantly improve their knowledge and skill not only by acknowledging their errors but by learning from them in an effort to improve themselves and their patient care. A professional will weigh the needs, benefits, and risks to patients, family, colleagues, and self in whatever he or she pursues; to do otherwise would be unprofessional or lack in professionalism.

With the development of more specialties and emphasis on productivity within dentistry, there is a risk of professionalism becoming depersonalized and centered on productivity in an impersonal system. There is a risk of no longer improving interpersonal communication but instead advancing an efficient commercial exchange. This may lead to the dentist healing the physical parts of the patient but not the whole person; the patient becoming a collection of parts treated by specialists. The very meaning of healing – that is, to make whole – may become lost. Therefore, dentists need to treat patients as people and not just another case of dentition to repair or to replace.

Learning Professionalism

Is professional behavior something innate, something you are born with, or is it something learned? It is most certainly something that can be learned. There are two ways by which one can learn professionalism: formally and informally.

Formally, professional behavior is taught in dental school not only as a course topic but also as what is expected of a dental student. Most dental schools, if not all, have a "white coat ceremony" in which the dental student is promoted into the profession. Courses are given on principles of dentistry and ethics, through various case scenarios. Patients are screened and appropriately placed with students, who follow standards to be followed by proper evaluation. Thus, a dental student is given ethical and professional concepts that he or she is expected to know, understand, and work within while treating selected patients. However, no matter how much classroom experience a dental student is exposed to, he or she will most likely learn and assimilate ethical professional behavior informally as well. A dentist as a professional should have a constant yearning to enhance his or her knowledge and skills, formally and informally, for the improvement of patient care, a true desire to avoid mediocrity.

The informal or hidden ways by which a dental student learns are through every influential faculty and staff member within a dental school. Dental students look up to their professors at all levels for guidance, not only in the technique protocols, but also in the proper professional behavior for various situations both within the school environment and outside it. Role modeling occurs whether or not the role model was intending to teach. The dentist's attitudes, mindset, moral stance, and hour-by-hour decision making about how to use one's time, with patients and in many other matters, even including how, what, and how much to feel, are observed by the student and imitated assiduously. Not all faculty and staff are aware that the behavior they are modeling is being learned by students. They may be modeling behaviors that students do not understand or are interpreting incorrectly. Therefore, professional behavior is most likely to be taught in this hidden, informal way.

The real challenge to professionalism is when there is a conflict within your personal level of professionalism. With the intrusion of insurance companies and corporate dental service organizations (DSOs), the dentist will possibly be put into a conflicting situation of patient welfare and dental insurance limitations or DSO policies that do not fulfill the dentist's level of professionalism. The decision will be hard pressed when the dentist is given an either do it this way or lose your participation with the dental insurance company and/or your job. To solve conflicts the dentist must professionally, ethically, and legally analyze the possible results as they relate to not only the patient but also to the dentist themselves.

Professionalism Boundaries

Professionalism in patient relationships have boundaries. The first step is to recognize the relationship and evaluate whether there is an imbalance of power such that one dominates the other by position and/or knowledge. The ADA Principle of Ethics and Code of Professional Conduct (ADA Code), 2 (G) states dentists should avoid interpersonal relationships that could impair their professional judgment or risk the possibility of exploiting the confidence placed in them by a patient. This also applies to family members or someone with decision-making authority for the patient. If the situation should arise, it is highly recommended to end the professional level of the relationship and allow for a cooling off period to eliminate any inferences of impropriety based on the dentist's position.

Being a professional, you should refrain from inappropriate behavior. The ADA Code 3 (F) states dentists have the obligation to provide a workplace environment that supports respectful and collaborative relationships for all those involved in oral health care. You should refrain from inappropriate comments that may be taken as flirtatious banter or tasteless jokes.

To maintain your professionalism, beware of any harassing behavior. There are many forms of harassment that once it is alleged, it is hard to defend. Besides sexual, verbal, and physical, there is also stalking, menacing, cyber-stalking, electronic, and creating or taking part in a hostile environment [4].

Many patients will ask for you to exchange business or to barter services and/or items. Beware that the exchange should be of fair market value, properly reported as income and that such quid pro quo could imply preferential treatment and/or question the dentist's objectivity.

Accepting patient gifts may be appropriate if it is merely an expression of appreciation and does not influence treatment or given to gain influential or inappropriate attention.

Many patients are involved in fundraising and will call upon you to donate a charitable contribution, which is fine. However, when the dentist solicits contributions from the patients, there are some guidelines that should be followed so as to not interfere with the doctor–patient relationship. It should not be done at the time of treatment such that the patient feels exploited by the imbalance of the situation. If you are so motivated to solicit donations from the patient, it must be done separately from the dental visit and not allude to preferential treatment.

With social media being a dominant communication pathway, your professionalism will be easily tested. Sites like Facebook, Instagram, Twitter, and LinkedIn easily blur the boundaries placed on professionalism. The Internet is a public venue, and once posted lives forever. The best advice is to keep your personal and professional lives separate and always monitor your postings. Keep in mind if whatever you post would make you feel uncomfortable if it were disclosed to a colleague or the public should not be posted.

Leadership

Professionalism also entails the quality of leadership. Leadership occurs not only within the dental practice, but also within the community where the practice is located. Leadership in a group often defaults to the higher educated professional within that group, due to the perception that the professional is better trained and therefore more knowledgeable. Thus, leadership within the community can fall on the dentist, being a professional with higher education. People automatically look to a doctor to act properly and professionally, regardless of the doctor intending to or not. Hence, you should always be aware of the social implications of being a professional and behaving responsibly, so as to act as a role model for others.

Leadership within the office is essential to a successful dental team and building a trusting doctor–patient relationship. Leadership entails the ability to gather information promptly and to make a decision or act accordingly with success. Employees require leadership for guidance to work together and be productive for the office. Without a leader, the practice would possibly function but not progress successfully. With a dentist with good leadership skills, the practice will become successful by bringing the employees together to form a dental team. Those skills should include writing a mission statement and a vision for the practice, fiscal responsibility, and proper business decision making.

Patients also need leadership qualities in their dentist. Not only must the dentist give treatment options to the patient per informed consent and patient autonomy, but the dentist must also ethically guide or lead the patient to a proper treatment plan through communication. Looking to the dentist for guidance, patients often base their treatment decisions on the recommendations of the dentist. However, care must be taken by the dentist not to impose his or her priorities on the patient without proper communication to educate the patient and to keep the patient's autonomy intact. More information on leadership can be found in Section 3 in "Leadership and Communication in Dentistry."

Therefore, the dentist/leader must have a positive, enthusiastic, can-do attitude to motivate and encourage employees and patients. This leads to a discussion of a "successful" dentist. Many point to financial accomplishments when defining success. Success, however, is much greater than the accumulation of wealth. Leaders are normally seen as successful people. But what is "success?" The letters spell out the definition:

Sense of direction by setting proper goals for themselves and others (patients, staff).
Understanding situations and people.
Courage to do the right thing.
Charity toward others in need.
Esteem in both professional and personal life.
Self-confidence by being informed and knowledgeable.
Self-acceptance by having an understanding of oneself [5].

The real test of professional ethical behavior is when a conflict of worthy values erupts and ethical decisions must be made. Simply being taught "to always be honest" or "to always be truthful" leaves a lot of room for faulty decision making and little to fall back on to help formulate a professional and fair ethical decision.

To summarize professionalism:

Practice Altruism – Put the patient's interest first at all time.
Respect and Responsibility – Treat others as you would like to be treated, take responsibility for all your actions, not just the good ones.
Open to All – Treat everyone without bias or prejudice, even if they differ from you.
Fidelity – Remember and honor the fact that patients and colleagues/staff both trust and put their confidence in you.
Empathy – Put yourself in your patient's shoes, remember to respect their perspectives to allow for excellence in practice.
Social Contract – We have a duty as professionals to respect the patient's trust in us, maintain competence and to inform them of the treatment we are doing and why we are proposing to do it.
Self-regulation – the cornerstone of being a professional, we must take this responsibility with utmost seriousness. If asked to participate in Peer Review, we must partake.
Integrity – Keep Ethics and Humanism as the core of your patient care philosophy.
Oath – Use the ADA Code and Oath of the Professional as a resource for guidance and centering in time of ethical question or challenge.
Never Stop Learning – Embrace life-long learning for the benefit of your patients. Competence is a core part of being a professional [6].
Attitude – Keep and maintain a positive attitude toward patients, staff, and colleagues.
Leadership – Take the initiative and step up to take part when asked to help.
Insight – Do not be afraid to offer your opinion or insight when asked.
Self-reflection – Take the time to develop your emotional intelligence and self-awareness.
Mindfulness – Be fully present and aware of your actions and where you are without judgment.

References

1 Jos Welie, "Is Dentistry a Profession? Part 1. Professionalism Defined," *Journal of the Canadian Dental Association*, Vol. 70, No. 8 (November 2004), p. 530.
2 David Ozar and David Sokol, *Dental Ethics at Chairside* (Washington, DC: Georgetown University Press, 2002), pp. 37–41.

3 Jos Welie, "Is Dentistry a Profession? Part 3. Future Challenges," *Journal of the Canadian Dental Association*, Vol. 70, No. 10 (November 2004), pp. 676–677.

4 Bruce Seidberg, "Harassment-Crossing the Professional Line," *Endodontic Practice*, Vol. 6, No. 5 (2013).

5 Maxwell Maltz, *Psycho-cybernetics* (Englewood Cliffs, NJ: Prentice-Hall, 1960), p. 113.

6 Julie Connolly, Task Force on Professionalism, *American College of Dentistry News*, Spring 2022, p. 5.

17

Ethics

Ethics is defined as "of or relating to moral action, conduct, motive or character; as ethical emotion; also treating of moral feelings, duties or conduct; containing precepts of morality; moral. Professionally right or befitting; conforming to professional standards of conduct" [1]. Decisions on which type of material to use or how to treat a certain situation are guided by treatment protocols. How to decide a fair, just disposition of an ethical situation or dilemma, however, will keep one up for nights. It is the dentist's responsibility and duty to maintain a professional demeanor that includes consideration, respect, and understanding toward fellow colleagues, employees, patients, and their families.

Ethics is about you and your interactions with others. It is how you make decisions and live with them because once a decision or choice is made it is yours forever. Who you are today is the result of all your thoughts, choices, and actions up till now. Who you will be tomorrow will be the result of your thoughts, choices, and actions of today. You are the one who fashions your life by what thoughts you hang on to, the choices you make, and the actions you take. Your ethical actions/choices are dependent on your last most dominant thought prior to that action or choice.

Becoming unethical is a slippery slope that is often times not recognized till it is infringing on yourself or others. The more one acts unethically, the easier to live with it and accept it as the norm. For example: Almost every house has the proverbial junk drawer where things are accumulated, or the back seat of the car where things just start piling up over time. In both cases, there comes a point where you cannot fit any more into the junk drawer before it won't close or the stuff in the back seat starts pouring over onto the front. Only you can stop the overflow and control how much to allow in the drawer or backseat. Likewise, ethics is the obedience to the unenforceable; such that, you correct yourself early to prevent sliding down the slippery slope.

The other pillars of decision-making must also be taken into consideration: dental law, risk management, and practice management (public relations) in your interaction with patients, staff, and your community. There are situations that will conflict between the pillars of decision-making.

Another area of concern in the discussion of ethics is how morals contribute. Morals constitute a basic human mark of right behavior and conduct, ethics are more like a set of guidelines that define acceptable behavior and practices for a certain group of individuals or society. They coexist in most situations.

Professional Responsibility in Dentistry: A Practical Guide to Law and Ethics, Second Edition. Joseph P. Graskemper.
© 2023 John Wiley & Sons, Inc. Published 2023 by John Wiley & Sons, Inc.

Code of Ethics

To gain a foundation from which the dentist may formulate thought and, it is hoped, a proper decision, the American Dental Association (ADA), FDI World Dental Federation, and many other groups have developed codes of ethics. These codes of ethics should guide the dentist in his or her decision making at all levels of practice, in one's professional career, and even in one's personal life. But, as will be pointed out, decision-making cannot occur in a vacuum, only considering the various codes of ethics.

Throughout these codes, the following principles may be found: patient autonomy, nonmaleficence, beneficence, justice, veracity, and fidelity.

Patient autonomy gives the patient, or the patient's legal guardian, the right to confidentiality and self-determination; in this case, the right to decide a course of treatment. Chapter 8 discussed the five levels of a patient's capacity to participate in that right to decide. The lower the level of capacity to understand, the more the dentist must take care in his or her informed consent to maintain patient autonomy. The dentist may be inclined or even forced to ask if the patient is in need of guardian-like help from friend or family (see True Case 25). Patient autonomy intersects with informed consent. Does the patient's incapacity compromise their autonomous decision making? Giving a proper informed consent with all relevant, necessary information for an informed decision is a major facet in the patient's right to self-determination and, hence, maintenance of patient autonomy. Patient autonomy also intersects with the doctor–patient relationship and the Health Insurance Portability and Accountability Act (HIPAA) in its principles of confidentiality. By respecting the patient's privacy to personal information, with the understanding that such personal information belongs to the patient and should not be made known to others without the patient's consent, the dentist is able to also adhere to a trusting doctor–patient relationship and HIPAA laws [2].

With the development of cosmetic dentistry, there has been an increase in the patient's awareness of his or her smile. Dentists also have promoted improving the patient's smile through cosmetic dentistry. The question becomes, "How much should a dentist pursue or promote the improvement of a patient's smile before the dentist is intruding into the patient's autonomy?" To keep the patient's autonomy intact, when the dentist perceives a cosmetic need, he or she must keep the discussion educational to properly inform the patient of cosmetic dentistry's capabilities. It should not become a commercial, merchant-like sale. Not all patients want nor have to have the perfect smile. Therefore, the dentist must not take advantage of an unsuspecting, unknowledgeable, trusting patient for the purpose of advancing the dentist's own well-being or income.

There is also the autonomy of the doctor to have the freedom to exercise their professional judgment in the care and treatment of their patients [3]. Dentists should have the autonomy in the manner of treating their patients from what materials, diagnostic tests and approved acceptable techniques and/or procedures that are available.

The limit of the patient's autonomy is self-injury, which brings us to the next principle of nonmaleficence.

Nonmaleficence is the principle that creates a duty to cause no harm to the patient. Nonmaleficence may be seen throughout the practice of dentistry. First and foremost, the dentist must know his or her limitations of practice and stay within those limitations and the standard of care. The dentist should avoid unlearned and experimental treatments without a true research-level informed consent. In attempting to try new procedures, the dentist must take the time and make the effort to be properly trained such that the risk of harm to the patient is at a minimum. It is clearly unethical to try an unproven treatment on an unsuspecting, trusting patient to whom the risk of harm is greatly increased. It is also the duty of the dentist to properly refer the patient when the needed treatment is beyond the dentist's capabilities. By referring the patient, the standard of care is also properly followed. In a situation where the patient refuses the referral, an informed refusal then takes place, as discussed in Chapter 8. This situation, as seen in True Case 42, becomes even more stressful for the dentist when the patient states, "Just do the best you can, Doc."

True Case 42: Patient doesn't want referral

A patient came to a dentist who was on her insurance company's list of participating dentists. The patient was in need of endodontics on a second molar with very curved, calcified canals, which already had a clinically viable porcelain-to-metal crown. When the dentist told the patient that he wanted to refer her to an endodontist, the patient became angry with the him, because he would not treat her; although she thought very highly of him. The dentist unsuccessfully tried to explain the complexity of the situation. The patient, on the other hand, told the dentist of the trust she had in him and that he had already successfully performed a root canal for her in the past. The dentist performed the root canal but was highly stressed, though it ended with a positive result. The result could have easily resulted in a bad outcome on many levels.

Law and ethics also intersect in the case of abandonment of a patient. Abandonment (See Chapter 11) of a patient, more times than not, results in injury to the patient due to delayed treatment; therefore, it is unethical. When a patient is under the care of the dentist, the dentist must take every precaution to cause no harm to the patient.

Harm is not only physical but may also be seen as emotional when personal relationships develop between dentist and patient. A personal relationship with a patient has long been frowned upon, due to the possibility of either party exploiting the relationship. It truly infringes on the patient's confidence in the dentist and impairs the dentist's professional judgment. Legally, it also can lead to alleged sexual harassment, which is not covered by malpractice insurance, as previously noted.

Nonmaleficence may also be found to be violated by a dentist promoting his or her experience as being more extensive than what it really is. A true informed consent concerning a procedure that is new to the dentist may not be found to be valid if the dentist did not inform the patient that it is a procedure new to the dentist and that he or she is doing it for the first time. This would obviously affect a reasonable person's autonomous decision-making.

True Case 43: I don't want my teeth

A patient needing extensive care, including periodontal surgery, extractions, endodontics, and restorative work, came into the dentist's office wanting to have all her teeth removed and dentures made because she was tired of all the pain and expense of treatment. She had previously undergone extensive treatment 10 years prior and did not wish to do it again. There were many easily saveable teeth that would have been excellent for partial dentures. The patient became adamant that all teeth should be removed. The dentist tried several different ways to explain that what she was requesting was not in her best interest. She then told the dentist to either see the situation her way or she would go elsewhere. The dentist proceeded to accommodate the patient. At the appointment to reline her immediate denture, the patient profusely cried that she should have listened to the dentist. The dentist felt very bad that he was not able to communicate better to help the patient understand the situation.

It may have been better for the dentist to refuse the patient, if a patient's autonomy extends to self-injury as seen in True Case 43. Ethically, but not legally following treatment protocols within the standard of care, the dentist should have thought about possibly denying the patient treatment.

Beneficence is the principle where the dentist has a duty to promote the patient's well-being. This can be easily seen in informed consent, treatment planning, and proper referrals. But it is also found in providing treatment in a timely manner regardless of the method of payment. Once a dentist has undertaken a procedure, he or she must proceed to a point in treatment so as to not cause harm, as discussed previously, but also to promote the well-being of the patient. This does not mean that treatment must be provided for free when the patient will not meet his or her agreed financial responsibilities. But the dentist must not ethically leave the patient in a worse condition. Hence, prior to starting any extensive treatment, a proper financial agreement and informed consent must be had, as discussed in Chapter 23. In promoting the patient's well-being, the dentist is ethically obliged to report any patient abuse – elder adult as well as child abuse. It should also be pointed out that legally, as discussed in Chapter 7, dentists are mandated to report suspected child abuse.

Dentists promoting dental or oral health care products should take great care not to take advantage of the doctor–patient relationship. The undue influence of a trusting patient to buy such products may not be in the patient's best interest. To alleviate any violation of beneficence, the dentist should not place pressure or obligation on the patient to purchase such products. In recommending such products, even though they may be beneficial to the patient, the dentist must take care in product promotion with any emphasis given to patient is based on the patient's needs and not on the need to buy the product to increase profits. Again, communication and education of the patient is paramount.

Justice is found in the principle of fairness. Dentists have the duty to treat all patients fairly. Dentists may not discriminate, be biased, or refuse treatment to a patient based on race, creed, color, sex, sexual orientation, disability, or national origin. Dentists should have a cross-cultural awareness and have respect for all cultures other than his or her own. As the saying goes, "Sharing is Caring." Hence, make a good faith effort to understand a patient's cultural view of health care to help build a trusting relationship. There are many antidiscrimination laws that also forbid such action.

This principle also needs to be followed in the treatment of patients with a lesser form of insurance than those who personally and fully pay for dental services (a self-paying patient). Just because a patient may have a lesser paying insurance, he or she should not be treated differently from those with better or no insurance. This does not mean that the lesser paying insurance patient is entitled to receive the same dental treatment, such as implants versus a partial denture, as a patient not relying on the insurance company to pay for the treatment. There are policy limitations that must be followed, and it is the patient's right to decide whether he or she will rely on the insurance, thereby only accepting treatment within those guidelines, being within the standard of care. All treatment options must be presented to all patients. In other words, those with poor paying insurance or welfare benefits should not be treated like second-class citizens, but should be treated equally and fairly as to the appointment time allotted, time spent, and standard of care provided. There should be no delay of treatment or limited access to appointments because the patient has a poor insurance reimbursement or payment. If there is a collision of profit making and fair treatment for all patients, the dentist would be ethically wise to reconsider his or her involvement in various dental insurance programs.

Veracity and fidelity principles go to the heart of the doctor–patient relationship, informed consent, and professionalism. Veracity is the principle of truthfulness when communicating with the patient, guardian, and others involved in the patient's treatment directly or indirectly. When critiquing previous treatment, be truthful, factual, understanding, and justifiable. Without truthfulness, the trust placed in the doctor–patient relationship would be a myth. It would also undermine dentistry's social contract with society, due to a loss of trust in dentistry as a profession because a dentist was not truthful. Veracity also goes to the image dentists portray to the public in the form of marketing or advertising. Many codes of ethics and state statutes address false and misleading advertising as being unethical and unlawful (see Chapter 21).

Fidelity goes hand in hand with veracity. This is the duty to keep one's word. This principle promotes professionalism by creating a duty to stand behind what he or she may say and/or do. In general, guarantees in the health care field are unethical and illegal in most states. However, it is entirely ethical to be a professional and stand behind or to be available when treatment ends in an unfavorable or unexpected result as seen in Ture Case 44. There are many situations in which fidelity enters the doctor–patient relationship that is based on trust. For example, if the dentist stated that he or she would apply the costs of a temporary procedure to the final treatment, the dentist should keep his or her word and do what was promised.

Veracity regarding a previous dentist's treatment poses ethical and legal situations that must be confronted. When prior treatment does not meet the standards of a subsequently treating dentist, care must be taken in how the situation is explained to the patient. The ADA Code of Ethics states: "Justifiable Criticism. Dentists shall be obliged to report to the appropriate reviewing agency as determined by the local component or constituent society instances of gross or continual faulty treatment by other dentists. Patients should be informed of their present oral health status without disparaging comment about prior services. Dentists issuing a public statement with respect to the profession shall have a reasonable basis to believe that the comments made are true." It also states that a dentist is obliged to report gross or continual faulty treatment via justifiable criticism [4]. What is justifiable criticism? "Meaning of Justifiable. Patients are dependent on the expertise of dentists to know their oral health status. Therefore, when informing a patient of the status of his or her oral health, the dentist should exercise care that the comments made are truthful, informed and justifiable. This should, if possible, involve consultation with the previous treating dentist(s), in accordance with applicable law, to determine under what circumstances and conditions the treatment was performed. A difference of opinion as to preferred treatment should not be communicated to the patient in a manner which would unjustly imply mistreatment. There will necessarily be cases where it will be difficult to determine whether the comments made are justifiable" [5]. Therefore, this section is phrased to address the discretion of dentists and advises against unknowing or unjustifiable disparaging statements against another dentist. However, it should be noted that, where comments are made that are not supportable and therefore unjustified, such comments can be the basis for the start of a disciplinary proceeding against the dentist making such statements.

Additionally, there is the risk of a defamation/slander lawsuit from the prior dentist. The absolute defense for defamation/slander is the truth. However, the time, effort, and costs involved in defending such a claim may prove to be burdensome. The courts look to the slandering remark as to whether it was a statement of fact or opinion. Courts have agreed that statements of opinion are not actionable. Therefore, when commenting on previous treatment by another dentist, start your statement with "In my opinion."

This is also the case when giving second opinions. Be very careful in criticizing the previously treating dentist. When commenting on the previous dentist's treatment, be fully aware of the respectable minority rule, as described in Chapter 12. Keep in mind that many times there is more than one way to treat a situation and more than one philosophy of treatment protocol that another dentist may follow or believe. Many treatment philosophies exist, all of which may be successful. Most dentists are ethically responsible professionals wanting to do their best for their patients. You also may direct the patient back to the previous dentist or offer to call the previous dentist to professionally discuss the difference of opinion. Most dentists will want to see what the situation is and correct it if it is needed. The patient may also be referred to the peer review board of the local dental society. Always remember that dentists are humans and everyone has a "bad hair day," so to speak, along with the fact that some patients are very difficult to work on. There is also the difference between bad dentistry and a bad result. Though the difference is not always clear, it should be understood that even though the previously treating dentists most likely treated within the treatment protocols and standard of care, the result was significantly less than ideal. So, before you have the thought that "I can do better," carefully evaluate the situation.

True Case 44: Fractured porcelain

A long-time patient needed a porcelain-to-metal bridge. It was the custom and habit for this dentist to tell patients after each visit to call if any problem occurs. All went well until two months after the bridge was cemented. The porcelain fractured in several areas. This could have occurred because the patient bit something hard or because the processing of the bridge was not ideal. Several different scenarios could have developed: Tell the patient "Tough luck, you broke it," and charge the full fee for a new bridge. Tell the patient to pay a percentage of the remake. Tell the patient that you would be happy to remake it at no charge, explaining that you are doing so to be as helpful as possible under the circumstances. Of course, the possible legal threat of a nuisance case, the practice management of public relations, and an unhappy patient will all play into the dentist's decision. The dentist in this case remade the bridge after consideration of the various possible outcomes and the ethical, legal, and practice management ramifications.

Teaching Dental Ethics

Ethics, like professionalism, is also taught outside the classroom. This teaching occurs through the observation of peers and colleagues, and, of course, how one has been brought up. There are also the cultural differences to be appreciated. What is thought to be proper in one culture may very well be avoided in another. Cross-cultural awareness should be respected to understand the patient's "dental IQ" and to properly educate and treat him or her. Nevertheless, all the major religions of the world have principles that refer to "doing no harm" (nonmaleficence), "making things better" (beneficence), "being fair" (justice), and "truthfulness" (veracity) [6]. Therefore, following these basic ethical principles, the dentist is able to reach out and understand the various cultures and beliefs that affect his or her providing optimum dental care for the patient.

Ethical choices are not always learned in a classroom but through experiencing ethical behavioral results of either your own choices or how others' choices have ethically affected you as seen in True Case 45. We become a product of those experiences. Hence, ethics is learned through the trial and error of ethical decisions that have either failed or succeeded, whether they are our own decisions or those of others that have had an impact on us. An ethical person strives to learn from the wrong decisions and repeat the right ones. As discussed in Chapter 16, one of the attributes of professionalism is the willingness to acknowledge errors and correct them when possible.

True Case 45: No pay, no treatment

A mother brought her eight-year-old son into the dental office because the boy, a new patient, was in pain. The dentist, a recent graduate, was an associate in a large practice. The owner dentist was always concerned about the payment for services. He was a true believer that no one should get free dentistry. The young associate examined the patient and informed the mother that a pulpotomy and stainless steel crown were needed. The mother stated that she did not have that much money, so the young dentist asked the owner dentist if he could just do the pulpotomy to relieve the pain. The owner dentist said no and that if he wanted to do free dentistry, he should find another job. The young dentist, feeling very badly, informed the mother that he was not allowed to do any treatment without payment. The mother and the boy left, understandably upset.

Ethical Challenges

There are many ethical issues in the earlier case regarding both the young dentist and the owner dentist. Ethically, but not legally, treatment should have been provided to relieve the pain. However, there is no legal duty to provide free dentistry.

The dentist's ethical integrity will be challenged on three levels:

1) Societal: Multicultural awareness will affect ethical decisions because some cultures outside the United States do not place as much value on dentistry. Patients with different cultural backgrounds may have preconceived, invalid notions that will be hard for the dentist to overcome and that will affect the patient's decision making. As society moves to more inclusive health care insurance, dentists will be tempted to seek insurance payment by manipulation of billing codes or service dates, for example. There will also be a change in dental health care values of the patient, due to their dependency on the insurance coverage. He or she will only consent to what will be paid by the insurance company, even if it is not the ideal treatment, for example, a covered extraction rather than root canal therapy, build-up, and crown. Society's emphasis on a perfect smile may push the dentist to incorrectly treat the patient's perceived needs, in other words, to allow the patient to direct the sequence of care; for example, treating the patient's perceived anterior cosmetic wants rather than treat the posterior rampant caries and the need of immediate care, though not visible to the patient. Here patient autonomy is stretched to a point where the dentist could be promoting the patient's self-injury by ignoring the patient's true needs.

2) Environmental: The intrusion of dental manufacturers, self-made dental gurus, and private dental continuing education institutions will affect the dentist in his or her choice of materials or treatment protocols. In addition, patients can easily access information outside the normal doctor–patient relationship via direct advertising from the manufacturer to the patient and via the Internet. With this partial and possibly biased information, the patient's expectations of infallibility of the technology, materials, and even the dentist's treatment may not be met.

3) Personal: The dentist must meet the expectations of his or her colleagues, staff, and family. These all place ethical and financial stresses on the dentist to meet expectations, competition, and responsibilities that, at times, may not be attainable unless the dentist bends an ethical concept or principle.

Other stressors on a dentist's ethics are more internal to dentistry's self-image. Are we losing our professionalism to the selling of dental appliances or prostheses by the promotion of "crowns in an hour," "teeth in a day," or "immediate bleaching"? These are all wonderful advancements in dentistry, but as their promotion becomes more merchant-like, does our professional image in society diminish? Are we changing from dental health care to "image care" or "self-esteem dentistry"? Of course, cosmetic dentistry has greatly helped many patients obtain a positive change, but will this, rather than the patient's well-being, become a primary goal? With more highly educated patients, are we headed toward fulfilling a patient's wants prior to his or her dental needs? Will the dentist become an agent of the patient, whereby the knowledgeable patients dictate treatment, making the dentist more of a hired craftsman?

There are situations that require a distinction of legal and ethical concepts when professional duty arises that is either ethical but not legal or legal but not ethical. There are many scenarios that bring this to point: legal refusal to treat a patient in pain, as seen in True Case 45, or ethically provide emergency treatment for a minor without an informed consent. For example, when the planned treatment extends beyond that which was originally planned and the parent or guardian cannot be contacted after a good faith effort, one should not legally proceed without proper informed consent; but ethically one should treat the patient and adhere to beneficence and nonmaleficence in the best interests of the patient. To help separate ethics and law in a simple nutshell: the law is what we should or must do and ethics is why we should do it or not do it.

Decision Making

In addition, many state laws (as discussed previously) affect the dentist's ethical behavior and decision making. So how does one properly apply not only ethical concepts but also legal rules and regulations and practice management guidelines when a decision must be made? Professional chairside decisions should be based on all facets of that which affects the dentist, the patient, the practice, and the profession. To do this, there are four basic steps to lead to a correct decision: Issues, Rules, Analysis, and Conclusion (IRAC):

1) What issues are presented ethically, legally, and professionally, through risk management and practice management?
2) What ethical concepts, legal rules or regulations, practice management and risk management guidelines, or responsibilities to the profession apply?
3) Assess and analyze all issues and possible decisions/results as they apply to all the interested parties or stakeholders in the decision.
4) Arrive at a conclusion as to the decision to be made or action to be taken.

Applying IRAC may be used as a discussion guide to the examples in the following chapter or to any of the True Cases.

References

1 Henry Campbell Black, *Black's Law Dictionary*, 5th Edition (St. Paul, Minn., West Publishing, 1979), p. 496.
2 John R. Williams, *Dental Ethics Manual* (Ferney-Voltaire, France, FDI World Dental Federation, 2007), p. 56.

3 Nobuya Hashimoto, *Japan Medical Association Journal*, Vol. 49, No. 3, 2006, p. 125–127. accessed May 20, 2022).

4 American Dental Association, *Principles of Ethics and the Code of Professional Conduct*, 2005, Section 4, 4.C.

5 Ibid., Section 4, 4.C.1.

6 Jeffery Moses, *Oneness Shared: Great Principles Shared by All Religions* (New York, Random House, 1989).

18

Professional Ethical Situations Based on True Cases

A patient comes into your office with a denture that is five years old and says, "My insurance will pay for a new denture every 5 years, so I'm here for my new denture." You have rent and payroll due, and it's been a slow month. You check the fit of the denture and it is satisfactory. The patient acknowledges no problem eating anything and thinks they look great. He only wants new dentures because the insurance will pay for them. He also has an old denture as a spare. The insurance company will pay only for needed treatment. However, the patient feels he is entitled to his new dentures since he pays all his premiums on time. What are you going to do?

You have just started a new job as an associate in an established, high-quality office. The employer/owner dentist has diagnosed four quadrants of scaling and root planning for the patient you are seeing. On checking the periodontal condition, you find no pocketing >4 mm with only slight supragingival calculus on the lingual of teeth #23 to #26. What are you going to say to the patient and to your boss, the employer/owner dentist?

The very next day you see another patient as the associate dentist. A tooth has been diagnosed by the employer/owner dentist to need a build-up and crown. On examination you find that a two-surface amalgam restoration, in your opinion, would function just as well. Your education loan payment is due and you really need this job. You are paid on a weekly production basis. What are you going to do?

A patient had a crown placed on #14. Two years later she comes in for a maintenance visit. The periodontal condition is within normal limits except between #14 and #15, where there is a 5 mm pocket and the tissue bleeds easily on probing. The patient states that she always gets food trapped between the two teeth ever since the crown was placed. Tooth #15 only needs an occlusal restoration. On examination, the contact between #14 and #15 is not ideal. In fact, it is open. What are you going to do? Extend the restoration on #15 to the mesial to tighten the contact even though there is no decay, or remake the crown on #14 (if so, at no charge or for some sort of reduced fee)?

A patient comes into your office with limited funds available for dentistry. He wants to do what is best. Tooth #18 has an old crown with slight marginal caries. Tooth #20 has a small occlusal amalgam with no caries. Tooth #19 is non-restorable. You recommend the extraction of #19. After talking with the patient, the patient says he can afford some treatment with a payment plan. Would you restore #18 and #20, and place an implant for #19, which would cost more because his insurance does not cover implant-related services, but would be ideal? Or would you make a bridge from #18 to #20, for which the insurance company would cover a portion of the payment and is within the patient's ability to pay, but would be less than ideal?

Professional Responsibility in Dentistry: A Practical Guide to Law and Ethics, Second Edition. Joseph P. Graskemper.
© 2023 John Wiley & Sons, Inc. Published 2023 by John Wiley & Sons, Inc.

Dr. Drillem is a provider in several insurance plans within a preferred provider organization (PPO), which include Save Teeth Dental Plan. He is not a member of the Always Smile Dental Plan. A new patient has coverage through both plans. Save Teeth Dental is the primary provider of insurance. On examination it was found that the patient has a crown that is loose, can be easily removed, and needs a replacement due to poor marginal integrity. After informing the patient of the need to replace the crown, the patient states that it is only eight months old and hoping it to be only recemented. Dr. Drillem's usual, customary, and reasonable (UCR) fee is $1000. Save Teeth Dental pays from a mutually agreed to, reduced fee schedule, whereby they pay 50% of a reduced fee of $600 for a crown less any deductible ($50 if not already paid) and/or any primary insurance benefit payment. Always Smile Dental Plan pays 50% of the reduced fee schedule, which allows $500 per crown less any deductible ($50 if not already paid) and/or any primary insurance benefit payment.

1) What should Dr. Drillem do about the crown only being eight months old? The preparation is non-retentive. It is very tapered and short.
2) Should Dr. Drillem discuss the quality of care with the patient?
3) Should Dr. Drillem contact the prior dentist?
4) Should Dr. Drillem contact the local dental society?
5) Is it truly bad work or merely a bad result? (As the doctor will find out, the patient is very difficult to work on due to limited access.)

Now consider Dr. Drillem is a member of both PPOs and the crown is over 10 years old.

1) What fees should Dr. Drillem charge?
2) What fees should he submit to each insurance company and what will be his total reimbursement?
3) How do things charge if the patient is over his yearly maximum?

Dr. Brand New went for an interview with Dr. Mega Practice, who employs several associates. During the interview, Dr. Practice explains to Dr. New that she will be paid a low base salary, and then on the production she does per month once she surpasses a certain goal. She is also informed that if a certain level of production, that which would cover her low base salary, is not made three months in a row, due to time constraints and the economics of the practice, she would be let go. Dr. Mega is a really nice person with a good reputation, and Dr. New has heard a lot of positive feedback from previous and current associates that if she works hard, she could earn a sizable income. Dr. New takes the job but is always running late with patients due to her effort to maintain quality in her work and proper care for the patients. Dr. New has lots of education loans and a car loan, and rent is due on her new apartment. The other associates tell her to just get it done as fast as possible because no one checks and that is how you make the money. What should Dr. New do?

Mrs. Cost made an emergency visit to Dr. Uptodate. Mrs. Cost is 72 years old and has been a very trusting patient of Dr. Now Retired, who sold the practice to Dr. Uptodate last year. Mrs. Cost has always taken care of her teeth with excellent home care and regular maintenance visits, because she did not have a lot of money. However, the last time Dr. Retired filled #5 with a large amalgam restoration, she remembers him telling her that someday it may need further work.

On examination, Dr. Uptodate found the lingual cusp and some of the mesial fractured off #5 (about one quarter down from where the cusp tip would have been). However, the old amalgam was intact and the pulp was not exposed. He also found no periodontal problem nor periapical lesion, and the tooth did not elicit a positive reaction to percussion, heat, or cold. Other than the chip, the tooth seemed to be sound. When Mrs. Cost smiles, her broad smile shows all the way back to the first molar. The facial aspect is completely intact and cosmetically acceptable.

Dr. Uptodate has renovated Dr. Retired's old office considerably with new equipment, including a completely computerized, digital radiographs, paperless office and patient record system, a scanning system, and a state-of-the-art laser. These renovations and equipment were very costly and the hefty monthly payments have become larger and more of a burden than Dr. Uptodate anticipated. Dr Uptodate is recently married and they are expecting a baby.

Dr. Uptodate thinks of the treatment options available, but also thinks about the bills to pay for the renovation and equipment, in addition to the purchase of the practice. He also has a small family to support. The options are an indirect pulp cap/bonded composite restoration (covered by insurance), root canal therapy/post (needed for the retention of the crown), all ceramic crown, a three-quarters coverage scanned and milled in-office restoration, or just to smooth it down. All the treatment options have an indication for use of the laser, but this increases the fees. Some of these options are longer lasting, some more ethical, and some covered by insurance.

Mrs. Cost has some funds for dentistry along with her dental insurance. Her insurance company will not pay for root canal therapy without apical pathology or laser. It will pay half of any of the other options.

1) What is Dr. Uptodate to do?
2) With the doctor–patient relationship in mind, how should Dr. Uptodate present his preferred treatment and why?
3) How hard should he sell, persuade, or influence Mrs. Cost?
4) Discuss legal responsibilities, ethical concerns, and decision-making affects on all parties involved.
5) What is legally and ethically at stake?

This last case is a combination of situations that may occur. There are many different practice philosophies and treatment protocols that can direct this scenario to many different outcomes, all of which have an impact on the patient and the doctor, personally and professionally.

Part IV

New Dentist Issues

19

Associateships

There are basically two types of associateships: employee and independent contractor. Both have legal and tax consequences. The type of associateship is usually determined by the employer as a condition of employment and is normally written in a contract signed by both parties. Some offices hire associates without a contract. It is highly advisable to have a contract to eliminate any misunderstanding between the associate and employer. The employer and the associate may delay drafting a contract for a few months to evaluate the future relationship. During that try-out period a short engagement agreement should be had detailing how the associate should be paid, if there is any restrictive covenant during the try-out, the associate's license and malpractice insurance are intact, and necessary information for proper insurance billing. However, it is advisable to wait no longer than 3–6 months to decide on a complete contractual relationship. It is preferable at the time of initial employment.

New dentists usually have three main concerns regarding their new associateship:

1) The Internal Revenue Service (IRS) view of their employment status.
2) The understanding of noncompete clauses/restrictive covenants.
3) The manner in which they will be compensated.

Although there are many facets to an employment agreement, only a few major concerns are addressed here. As always, legal advice should be had prior to signing any legal document, including employment agreements.

For many years there was a 20-item checklist that indicated the associate's status as an employee or independent contractor [1]. This checklist was very restrictive in allowing the independent contractor status and was left to the subjective opinion of an IRS agent. This has been replaced by an 11-part assessment that is divided into three categories: behavioral control, financial control, and type of contractual relationship [2]. The associate's status is very important, especially to the employer, because of the tax consequences. If the associate is an independent contractor, the employer does not have to withhold nor pay various payroll withholding taxes. The burden falls on the independent contractor to properly pay such taxes on a quarterly basis. The employer must, on the other hand, pay the taxes associated with an employee.

Behavioral control can be evaluated by the instructions given to an associate as to when, where, and how to perform his or her job duties. Many of the behavioral controls are intrinsic to doing dentistry. The new dentist usually does not have any control over the equipment or supplies he or she uses, the dental assistant, and dental hygienist assignments. These are under the employer's control. However, the associate dentist should have control over what work is performed and the

Professional Responsibility in Dentistry: A Practical Guide to Law and Ethics, Second Edition. Joseph P. Graskemper.
© 2023 John Wiley & Sons, Inc. Published 2023 by John Wiley & Sons, Inc.

order or sequence of that work. In other words, the associate should have some control over the patient's treatment plans, the sequence of the dental care proposed, and possibly the materials used. The more control the employer has over the associate, the less likely the associate is an independent contractor.

Financial control can be evaluated by the associate's possible realization of a profit or loss. This is balanced by the associate's having an investment with non-reimbursable expenses. In other words, does the associate have some control over his or her overhead? At first look, most associateships will not fulfill this category. However, on closer evaluation, this category may be fulfilled by having the associate pay portions of lab fees, implant supplies, setting his or her own fee usual, customary and resaonable (UCR) fee schedule, and/or certain office expenses, such as a dental assistant. Financial control is also evaluated by the manner in which the associate is paid. Being paid based on collection or production also shows that the associate has some control over his or her profit or loss. Collection or production compensation allows the associate more financial control than a per diem or hourly wage. The associate may form a S Corporation or a Limited Liability Corporation (LLC) setting up the possibility for the employer to hire the associate through the associate's corporation. This also gives the associate added legal protections plus the benefits of being incorporated. Prior to doing so be sure to check with proper legal and tax professionals within your jurisdiction.

The type of relationship is normally stated in the employment contract, such as employer–employee or employer–independent contractor. The contract should also clearly state, among other things, any benefits provided, how long the intended relationship is to last, and the responsibilities of each party. This should include the associate's access to patient records after employment if the need arises in defense of a lawsuit. The more benefits provided, the more likely the associate is to be acting as an employee. The length of employment is usually clearly stated in the contract of employment. The influence of the associate normally affects the noncompete/restrictive covenants, by the number of days working in the practice: the more the associate is working in the practice, the more the associate has influence within and on the practice.

Noncompete/Restrictive Convenants

Noncompete/restrictive covenants limit the time and distance an associate may practice while at the practice, and possibly after he or she leaves a practice, whether one is an employee or an independent contractor. These types of agreements protect the employer dentist from an associate quitting the practice, opening a practice nearby (as seen in True Case 46 and True Case 47), or becoming employed by a nearby dental office, and promoting him or herself in the attempt to take patients away from the previous employer. An employer who has spent 20 or more years building a practice runs the risk of losing it without such a covenant; hence the need for a restrictive noncompete agreement. As with any contract, there must be consideration as described in Chapter 4. The continuance of an at-will employment can be considered sufficient consideration [3]. Often the time is set in years during which one may not practice within a set distance from the employing practice. There is no set amount of time that is common in such an agreement. Nevertheless, the time clause must be legally reasonable. For example, if the associate works only half a day per week in a practice and the restrictive agreement time clause refers to a time period of five years after leaving employment, it will most likely be found to be unreasonable depending on your jurisdiction. The distance may be set in miles or specified by names of nearby towns based on the practice's range of influence or from where the practice draws patients. To be reasonable, the demographics surrounding the practice must be taken into account. A distance of 15 miles may be found to be too small in a very rural area; it may be found to be too large in a metropolitan area. The restrictive covenant should take into account the amount of time the associate works in the practice on a weekly basis and total length of time employed. As the associate's time increases in the practice, the restrictive covenant should become longer in time and wider in distance, but not become unreasonable. The level of competition around the practice and the associate's future employment opportunities are also taken in consideration in deciding the reasonableness of the restrictive covenant. Restrictive covenants may also state that the associate upon leaving is not allowed to treat those patients that may follow the associate. There may also be a clause restricting the solicitation of other employees or staff. The restrictive covenant is understandably more restrictive with the sale of a practice.

True Case 46: Dentist reopened next door

A dentist worked in a practice as an associate for about five years, after which he purchased the practice from the owner who was going to retire. Approximately a year after he bought the practice, the "retired" dentist opened a practice next door to the one he just sold. There was no restrictive covenant to prevent the "retired" dentist from opening the new practice. Due to the severe impact on the sold practice, a lawsuit was commenced.

True Case 47: Dentist takes all patient records to new office

A dentist worked three years as an associate in a large pedodontic/orthodontic practice; he was the orthodontist. The orthodontist routinely requested an employment contract and a purchase agreement from the owner dentist. Constantly being forestalled, the associate took all the orthodontic records and moved them into another office in which he worked part-time and began to work on opening his own office nearby. Lawsuits were filed.

In both of these true cases, the patients were confused as to where to place their trust and go for treatment. Hence, most contracts also have clauses referring to the ownership of the dental records and possible restriction of the associate's access to the records. Ownership of the records is normally with the owner or dental corporation per the written contract. As previously mentioned, the associate, via his or her employment contract, should have access to patients' files, even after leaving the practice, in case of a lawsuit.

Trade Secrets

In many contracts the associate is prevented from using "trade secrets." Trade secrets are "the formula, pattern, device, or compilation of information which is used in one's business and which gives one opportunity to obtain advantage over competitors who do not know or use it" [4]. It is any information that is not generally known to the public that confers some type of economic benefit on the owner of such confidential information who has taken a reasonable effort to maintain its secrecy. This refers to the manner in which the employer dentist runs the business of his or her practice, patient information, billing practices, but not the way dental procedures are done because that attaches to the dentist performing the treatment. From employee relations to practice promotion, patient information, the business model and any other information regarding the owner's business is protected. Traditionally, an employee has the right to quit but are prevented from taking trade secrets; and, independent contractors have the right to work elsewhere but not prevented from taking trade secrets unless there is a confidentiality agreement. Normally associates whether an employee or an independent contractor will need to sign a confidentiality agreement to protect the owner's interests.

Compensation

The biggest concern to most new dentists is how they will be compensated. There are many formulas available to compute an associate's compensation. There are basically three ways to formulate the associate's pay:

1) A percentage of collection
2) A percentage of production
3) Per diem or daily wages.

Sometimes the compensation may be a combination of the three concepts.

A percentage of collection is the most complex, in that records must be kept more carefully. There must be an understanding of how a patient's payment is applied to all the doctors involved. Most times the patient payments are applied to the oldest running balance. Hence, the associate must be fully aware of the practice's collection percentages. The associate must also keep records of his or her production and balance it with the collections or accounts receivable for each patient he or she sees. For proper accounting, the associate must rely on the owner dentist to provide an account receivable for each patient seen. Most practice management software makes such information easily available. The accounts should be reviewed by both on a monthly or quarterly basis depending on the associate's part- or full-time status.

Obviously, it is easier to compute compensation by using a percentage of production. It is easy for the associate to simply keep track of the work he or she has done for the day. With the fee schedule in hand, the associate only needs to figure the amount of production for each day. This will become more confusing if there are many insurance plans with reduced fee schedules that would require an adjustment to the UCR production fee. Again, most practice management software is able to easily compute the production, including the reduced fee schedule adjustments, on a daily basis.

Per diem or daily wages are when the associate is paid a set wage for the day, based on an eight-hour day. The associate is then relieved of overseeing the production and/or collection for the patients he or she has seen.

It is to be expected that payment based on the percentage of collection should be slightly higher than the percentage of production to accommodate some of the non-payment situations that occur when being paid on the total production amounts. The level of insurance involvement must be carefully evaluated for the true amount of compensation. If the insurance fees are low and the amount adjusted off the UCR fee is high, the percentage of the remainder or true payment may be unreasonably low. Hence, in such a situation to maintain sustainability, payment should be based on collections.

Many employment agreements have clauses that state what the associate will be financially responsible for, such as lab fees or implant supplies. If such a clause exists, review it carefully to establish its fairness. Normally, the percentage the associate is responsible for is the same percentage he or she receives as compensation.

Regardless of the manner in which the associate is compensated, the employment contract should be completed within 3–6 months of employment. If there is an opportunity to purchase some or all of the practice, it is highly advisable to seek a buy/sell agreement or letter of intent that describes the cost and manner of purchasing the practice. If there is a delay of one or two years before discussing the purchase of the practice, the associate may end up paying for the increase in practice value due to his or her endeavors and influence on the practice like what happened in True Case 48. Hence, the associate will pay more. It is better for the associate to obtain an equity position within the practice sooner, if such a relationship is intended.

True Case 48: Buy what you built?

An energetic, young new dentist was hired by the employer dentist to work evenings and weekends. There were two other associates already in the practice. The associate was told that if he "built up" the evenings and weekends, then he could then expand into more days. He was also told that if he became busy enough and his production matched that of the owner dentist, he would have the opportunity to buy into the practice. At the end of a year, the associate had grown the practice to accommodate full-time employment, and his production surpassed the owner's. The practice actually more than doubled in that one year and the other associates left. He approached the owner to purchase into the practice. He was told the total cost of the practice, and was offered the purchase of one half. Looking back at that purchase years later, the associate realized that he actually purchased the part he had grown. He should have had an agreed-upon purchase price prior to working hard and developing the practice further.

Due to the large education loans that many new dentists have, it may be best to compensate the associate in a variety of ways. With both, a set per diem and a production level, as seen in True Case 49, that must be met for additional compensation, the associate not only has a reliable income but also an incentive to be productive for the practice.

True Case 49: Earn your pay

A dentist hired an associate to increase the hours the office was open and to help in the rapidly growing practice. The new associate was given a very fair per diem. After each month the owner dentist would check and balance the production of the new associate with wages paid. It was found that the associate was costing more than the wages paid. The owner dentist was actually losing income by having an associate who had no incentive. On review of the cases with which the associate had been involved, it was found that the associate never discussed sealants for pedodontic patients and never discussed replacing missing teeth even when he extracted them unless they were in the anterior area. It became obvious to the owner that the associate was happy with not having to work and getting a set wage. This also raised questions about the diagnostic abilities of the associate as well as many ethical issues relating to beneficence and nonmaleficence. The associate was let go.

It is important that the associate keep records of production or collection and insist on a monthly or quarterly review to accommodate any needed adjustments.

Other concerns that must be recognized are "hold harmless clauses" (explained in Chapter 3), vacation time, sick days, maternity leave, handling after-hours emergencies, use of the associate's name in marketing, type of malpractice coverage, and continuing education expenses.

There are many different business settings with which an associate will be in contact. Some associates, never wanting the ownership of a practice and only "wanting to do the dentistry and go home," may also find it necessary to set up a business entity for themselves. The six major entities are:

1) Sole proprietor
2) Partnership
3) "C" corporation (professional corporation [PC])
4) "S" corporation
5) Limited liability partnership [LLP]
6) Limited liability corporation [LLC] (professional limited liability corporation [PLLC]).

Each of these entities has different legal exposures, tax liabilities, and benefits. It is beyond the scope of this book to fully discuss the benefits and risks of each entity. Briefly, the sole proprietor is the simplest form, whereby the dentist works for him or herself without any corporate legal protections. The partnership perhaps carries the highest liability, whereby each partner is fully liable for the other partner's actions. With proper construct, the corporation is the most common business entity for dentists. The LLC and the "S" type of corporations are most common due to the pass-through of income to avoid double taxation, as compared with a "C" corporation that is taxed on its income and again on the dentist's income. It is obvious that any dentist seeking to set up a business entity must seek proper legal and tax advice.

These business entities may also be found in various combinations when multiple owners are involved. The solo-group practice is such an entity where each dentist is a separate entity and all have a mutual agreement to share certain aspects of the practice, such as rent, supplies, equipment, and other office overhead under another jointly shared entity. Again, proper legal and tax advice is paramount.

Dental Service Organization (DSO)

Many dentists are hesitant to purchase a practice due to the expense and the large student debt that must be paid. Some dentists are not interested enough in the business of dentistry to be entrepreneurial and buy a practice or start a practice. As the saying goes, "The sooner you start, the sooner you finish". The same goes for becoming involved in corporate dentistry.

A dental service organization (DSO) is different from a private office associate contract which may nor may not buy the practice. It may only manage the practice for the dentist who may retain ownership. The DSO may purchase the practice with the selling dentist becoming an employee of the DSO. Therefore, the dentist loses any authority over the running of the practice. In consideration of working with or for a DSO, be aware of the following:

1) Time constraints and production quotas.
2) Has oversight of staffing that may lead to hiring lower paid, less competent staff.
3) Change materials, equipment, and dental labs to save money.
4) Will change fee structure, billing, insurance documentation to fit their format.

5) May use your name for billing insurance, which if found to be fraudulent, you will be held liable and not the DSO, which is called doctor identity theft. (If your name is on it, you own it!)
6) Office policies will change to match other DSO locations.
7) Control scheduling, informed consents, follow-up policies and access to after-hours care.
8) Controls how complaints, problems, and financials are handled. Complaints to the dental board or a malpractice claim will be held against the dentist and not the DSO corporation. A patient may have a complaint and you, the dentist, may never hear about it until it becomes a legal issue.
9) Social media comments and reviews usually attach to the dentist and not the DSO.
10) Type of malpractice insurance (occurrence or claims-made) and the consent to settle may be decided by the DSO. May not cover volunteer situations.
11) Any settled claim reported to the National Practitioner Data Bank will be made in the dentist's name and not the DSOs.
12) Hold harmless clause needs to be for both the dentist and the DSO, otherwise the DSO will have no liability.
13) May have clause to penalize dentist if he or she leaves prior to end of contract.
14) Restrictive covenants may cover other DSO owner locations and even possibly future locations.

For more information on DSOs and PPOs see Section 1 of "Leadership and Communication in Dentistry."

Key points to remember:

1) Do not tie yourself up with an unreasonable restrictive noncompete clause.
2) You should have a written employment contract within no more than six months of being employed. The sooner the better.
3) Keep your own records to verify wages, if paid on production or collections.
4) If interested in the purchase of the practice, try to secure a buy/sell agreement or letter of intent as soon as possible.

Always seek proper legal and tax advice prior to signing any contract or when necessary.

References

1 Joseph P. Graskemper, "The Wonderful World of the Independent Contractor," *Dental Economics* (November 1995), p. 75.
2 Peter Sfikas, "IRS' New Test," *Dental Practice Report* (May 2007), p. 54.
3 Zellner, v. Stephen D. Conrad, M.D, P.C., 589 N.Y.S. 2nd 903 (N.Y. App.Div.1992).
4 Henry Campbell Black, *Black's Law Dictionary*, 5th Edition (St. Paul, Minn.: West Publishing, 1979), p. 1339.

20

Starting or Buying a Practice

As with any business, it is often said that the three most important aspects are location, location, location. Everyone enjoys convenience and easy accessibility when taking care of life's needs; that includes going to the dentist. The location, whether you are buying a practice or starting a new practice, should have good visibility, be easily accessible, and have ample parking. Once leases have been signed and the equipment purchased, a bad location is hard to overcome. There should also be a good understanding of what signage is available to show where the practice is located as seen in True Case 50.

True Case 50: Do you see me now?

A new dentist decided to start his own practice in an office building that had space available on the second floor. He signed the lease, constructed the office, purchased the equipment, and was ready to place a small professional sign on the outside. On questioning the owner of the property, he was told there was no signage available and he would not have access to the building's sign in the front of the building. Signage rights were not included in the lease!

Therefore, be sure not only to seek legal and tax advice but also to confer with a practice management consultant familiar with dentistry to start your career on a great first step.

Location

To find the right location, the first and foremost thought is, where do you want to live? This does not mean that you have to live right next door to the practice, but consider your commute time. Consider rural, suburban, or city environments as to where you want to live and what type of practice you would prefer. Rural and suburban areas lend themselves to a greater involvement of the dentist in the community and closer personal ties to the patients as seen in True Case 51. In such areas the dentist will normally work, live, play, and pray in the same or a nearby community, whereas the larger the city, the lesser the community involvement and personal ties with the patients. You may also find demographic studies helpful in locating the right community. Demographic studies may be found at the local chamber of commerce, real estate offices, and possibly the local dental society. The studies should show generalized information regarding the area's population, such as average income, average cost of housing, and average age. Then

Professional Responsibility in Dentistry: A Practical Guide to Law and Ethics, Second Edition. Joseph P. Graskemper.
© 2023 John Wiley & Sons, Inc. Published 2023 by John Wiley & Sons, Inc.

consider the type of practice you want and whether you want to buy a practice, start a practice, or work as an associate.

True Case 51: You can run but you can't hide

A dentist decided to open a practice in a small village after selling his previous practice in a large city location. He did not realize that living in the village in which he practiced had some pluses and minuses. On the plus side, almost everyone knew who he was, even if they were not patients. This meant that every time he was in the village to buy groceries or go to the local pharmacy, he would see some patients. He had to be aware of his professional behavior at all times. On the minus side, he would have to accommodate intrusions into his personal time. While in line at the local bank, a patient confronted him regarding a statement that the patient thought was wrong, thinking he was charged twice for the same thing. This was quite a different situation from the dentist's previous large city practice, where he had a 45-minute commute.

Transfer/Setup Considerations

Besides location, there are many other facets to consider in the transfer of a practice. The details of the various types of transfer and factors involved are beyond the scope of this book, but there are some common concerns. In the consideration of whether to buy a practice, major concerns may include:

1) Whether all state and local code requirements and regulations have been met.
2) The condition of the equipment.
3) The condition of the office design and interior.
4) Whether the staff will stay.
5) Whether the income of the practice will cover the purchase payments, personal income, and any needed renovation.
6) Whether the lease can be transferred and/or renewed.
7) How many new patients per month lets you know if it is a growing practice.
8) Are the recall, collections, and insurance processing active and up-to-date.
9) To what extent is the practice involved in various insurance programs.

Depending on the location of the practice, some of the codes that must be met are sanitation, health department, fire safety, and federal handicap access codes. Failure to fulfill any of the codes may cause not only fines and penalties, but possibly closure of the office. With the change in ownership, a surprise inspection may uncover the necessity of costly changes.

The equipment of an existing practice must be evaluated by a trained repair person or other person capable of determining its condition and longevity. If you are not already working in the practice, it is highly advisable to work there a few days to determine whether you are able to use the existing equipment, to check the operatory layout and available dental supplies, and to observe the staff interaction.

Many times, when a practice is being sold, the selling dentist has not renovated the office for several years. Depending on the size of the office, painting and reflooring can be very costly. The need to renovate and the costs involved must be determined before any purchase price can be agreed on.

When a new dentist purchases the practice, the staff often becomes a critical factor. If the staff has been working there awhile and knows many of the patients on a more personal level, it is highly advisable to try and keep as many of them as possible. Try not to change office policies or staffing for at least six months so as to allow the patients to become adjusted to the new dentist. The typical introduction letter that you should send to the patients is usually not enough to convince patients to stay with the practice. The transition is much easier with a familiar staff supporting the transfer of the practice to the new dentist. As time progresses, adjustments to staffing may be achieved slowly without much impact on the practice.

For an active growing practice, 15–20 new patients per month is necessary to have continued growth. Of course, in areas of rapid growth, the new patients per month should be much higher when compared to a rather older established community with little change in demographics.

It is very important that the practice's various systems are active and up-to-date. There are many outside service companies that specialize in contacting patients for appointment reminders and recall maintenance visits. If such a service is being utilized, is it being overseen and followed up properly by the staff to make sure no patients are lost? There must be an active collection system within the practice to follow-up on patient's delinquent in their payments. Although it may just be a few patients in the category, they must be held accountable for any balances due. Most offices are now submitting insurance billing electronically. With the dental insurance industry being slow to pay or simply denying covered services, close oversight of insurance percentages being paid in a timely manner and patients' payment portions are collected correctly. Other considerations are setting production goals, adjusting the payroll scale, ordering policy and patient cancelation/no show policy.

The extent of insurance involvement is very important because it will have direct impact on your practice income. There should be a good mix of self-pay patients, preferred provider (PPO) patients, and in-office dental plan. Depending on the demographics, some practices may have a higher percentage of PPO patients. In that case be sure to check the amount of involvement in lower paying plans. It is not easy to simply stop accepting the plans without some plan to replace those patients that depend on that low paying insurance plan. More information on insurance involvement can be found in Section 1, "Leadership and Communication in Dentistry."

As with any major purchase of a business, the buyer must have enough capital to allow for income and unexpected needs. Therefore, you need to review the past and present practice finances. You will need to review the past three years and the most recent year to date Profit and Loss Statement and Balance Sheet. The Balance Sheet shows the assets and the liabilities of the practice. It only states what was paid for the asset and what the practice agreed to pay the banks to have the asset on that date. The Profit and Loss Statement is a financial statement that summarizes the revenues, costs, and expenses incurred during a specific period of time. It can be had for monthly, quarterly, six-monthly or yearly and also year-to-date intervals. There can also be a year-to-year comparisons that can give information on how the practice to growing. These should be reviewed with a Certified Public Accountant (CPA) who is familiar with dental practices to understand the financial position of the practice and understand income basis of accrual or modified cash, historical costs, depreciation, long and short term assets and liabilities, retained earnings, and owner's equity. These are all very important to realize your ability to have an income and repay the business bank loans used to purchase the practice. So, when applying for a loan, be sure to request enough money not only to cover the cost of the purchase but also to act as working capital to start you in the right direction.

Last and perhaps most important is to obtain a copy of the practice's existing lease to make sure it is transferable and renewable. If the selling dentist is the owner of the building, there should also be consideration of possibly buying the building in the future. This issue needs to be addressed for future wealth building. Unexpected situations may occur as seen in True Case 52. Owning your own office space is a bigger expense but increases your net worth. Leasing costs will always go up. There are many different types of leases. It can range from a full service lease where the landlord pays for all building support, utilities, insurance, maintenance, taxes to a single, double, or triple net lease where at each level the lease holder takes on more maintenance and tax responsibility ending with the triple net lease holder paying for all expenses of the office/building including taxes and insurance.

True Case 52: Poof! You're moving

An endodontist had a practice at the same location for over 20 years. It was in a great location in a small building that had three other small professional offices. The owner of the building decided to sell the building. The tenants were not notified until after the sale was completed. The new owner then said that all tenants must find new locations because he was going to use the entire building for his business. The tenants wished they had a "right of first refusal" or "option to buy" clauses in their contracts that would have allowed them to obtain the building by meeting any legitimate purchase offer.

As can be seen from this short discussion, you must have good advice from an attorney, accountant, and practice management consultant to properly purchase a dental practice or buy into an existing practice. With all factors being even, whether you start a practice or buy an existing practice, 5–7 years later the outcome is purely individual and usually equally financially successful.

Show Me the Money

Now that the right practice has been found in the right location, purchase money must be secured. There are basically three types of lenders: banks, private lenders, and Small Business Administration (SBA) loans. All of these lenders look to your ability to repay the loan. Banks are normally very friendly when lending money to professionals. Many banks may ask for a business plan to substantiate the loan. Private lenders usually have a higher interest rate and often will set up the purchase as a lease on equipment. Be aware of any lease that does not allow prepayment without a penalty and those with a prepayment that is merely a sum total of the lease payments, which already included the interest. To circumvent a future lease payoff problem, when another loan with lower interest rate becomes available, secure a payoff amount on a yearly or bi-yearly term at the time of signing the lease. Prior to applying for a business loan, review your credit score and cancel any unneeded credit cards (such as MasterCard, Visa, or department store cards). Also be sure to be current on all due loan balances. This will strengthen your position to acquire funds.

If a business plan is requested by the lender, it should contain the following nine aspects:

1) Business description: Describe what you are planning to do (general dentistry, specialty).
2) Market analysis: Describe the need for your services.
3) Product analysis: Describe what services you are planning to provide your patients (general dentistry, orthodontics, implants, etc.).
4) Competition: What other dentists in the vicinity offer and how your practice may differ.

5) Marketing strategies: How you plan to make people aware that you are there.
6) Operation: How many employees are needed and how the business is going to work.
7) Management: Describe who you are and what your credentials are.
8) Financing: How much money you need and how are you planning to use it.
9) Supporting information: Tell the lender any additional information to help the lender to get to know you and understand what you plan to do. If it is a new practice you are starting, the lender may also ask to have an accountant produce a "business forecast or projection" to see how the financial growth of the practice will take place [1].

When you seek a loan, other information will be required of you. Typically, the lender will require a personal financial report and copies of your past two years of federal tax returns. The personal financial report is basically a list of your assets less your debts, which equal your net worth. Lenders know that at the beginning of your dental career, the net worth will not be much and maybe even negative due to school loans. Be aware of acceptable debt and unacceptable debt. Acceptable debt attaches to education and anything that has a positive cash flow or the potential to increase one's net worth. It has appreciating value. Unacceptable debt attaches to cars, vacations, and credit cards and anything else that has a negative cash flow or lowers one's net worth. It has depreciating value.

Suggestions to lessen debt would be:

1) Always pay more than the minimum.
2) Pay off the highest interest loan/lease/credit card first.
3) Roll over high interest balances to lesser interest (0% credit cards, home equity, business line of credit).
4) Refinance higher loans by changing banks for lower percentages.
5) Avoid multiple credit card applications.

Credit scores are easily found. Many lending sources look to the FICO Score. Your FICO score is made up by the following:

35% payment history
30% amounts owed
15% length of history
10% new card inquiries
10% types of credit cards [2]

This information is necessary to eliminate those who have been irresponsible in their accumulation of early debt. Remember, your degree and potential to earn and pay back the loan is highly regarded. It is more efficient to apply to several lenders at the same time so as to not waste time, as the dentist did in True Case 53. This will give you a better negotiating position in seeking the best terms.

True Case 53: Bankrupt

A young dentist sought financing to purchase a large and successful practice. The dentist went to seven banks, only to be told by six of them that financing was not available. At one small bank, the bank president actually told the young dentist that he would be bankrupt if he were to buy the practice. Finally, on the seventh attempt, a bank agreed to finance the young dentist, who subsequently doubled the size of the practice within five years. As a side note, the bank that told him he would be bankrupt actually went bankrupt itself! The lesson here is: Never give up on a dream.

When setting up a new office or purchasing an existing practice, attention must also be paid to the percentages of overhead that will be encountered. If you are a new owner, marketing/advertising/promotion should be more than the average 3–5%. It is recommended to increase the marketing to 7%–10% for at least the first six months to bring attention to and introduce the new practice or new owner. There are many recommended spending percentages available for a practice to be successful. When starting or buying a practice, attention should be given to the difference of fixed and variable overhead expenses. A general list of normal expenditures with approximate percentages may be as follows:

Payroll (not including the dentist – somewhat variable)	**25%**
Lab fees (variable)	8%
Rent/utilities (fixed)	5%
Marketing (variable)	5%
Office/dental supplies (variable)	6%
Miscellaneous/insurance (variable)	3% [3]

As shown, the overhead could be approximately 52%. Any difference is directly related to your personal income. Therefore, throughout the lifetime of the practice, attention must always be paid to the overhead, especially the variable expenses, to maximize your income.

Balance Sheet and Profit and Loss

Professionally and ethically, you as a practice owner are responsible for the success of your practice. You must know how to understand the financial standing of your practice to provide not only care for your patients, but also provide a successful practice that can maintain payment of overhead and wages. Therefore, regardless of how big or small your practice is, you must have a balance sheet and a profit and loss statement. Banks use these reports to determine the strength of your business because it shows the assets and the liabilities of the practice. The balance sheet does not state what the practice is worth. It only states what was paid for the asset and what the practice agreed to pay to the banks to have the asset on that date. It is no more than a financial snapshot of your practice.

Assets are any valuable resources owned by the practice. There is long term (not to be converted to cash within a year), short term (will be converted to cash within a year) and intangible assets (that which was paid for such as trademarks, copyrights, or a phone number). Historical costs are the amounts paid for an item that incurred a debt and will be paid over time. Most times that is larger dental equipment (chairs, scanners, etc.).

The income of a practice can be accounted for under accrual basis (income is recognized when earned regardless of when collected) or modified cash basis (income is recognized when money is received). Dental practices use a modified cash basis due to all the adjustments that must be made and the number of patients that may be paying over time. There are also retained earnings that reflect the amount of profit (which is an asset) that was earned by the business since its beginning minus the money that was taken out or distributed to the owner(s). It is not the amount of cash that is in the bank. For example: The practice earns a profit and takes some of the cash to purchase an asset (equipment) or payoff a liability (loan for equipment), that equipment becomes retained earnings being fully paid off. If it is a loan, the equipment gains retained value as the loan is paid down. The ownership of the equipment moves from bank to practice owner as the loan is paid off.

The owner's equity is the amount of money (down payment) that the owner put into the practice from personal funds. The difference of what is owned and what is owed in the practice belongs to the dentist.

Expenses are reported as they are incurred. As with assets, there are long-term liabilities and short-term liabilities. Depreciation is the process by which the historical cost of a long-term asset loses bank/loan value over its useful life. So, the cost can be spread of a number of years. Per the jurisdiction and the constantly changing tax rules, the item purchased may be better to take a one-time full deduction for the item purchased.

The following are examples of a Balance Sheet and a Profit and Loss Statement.

Balance Sheet

Assets	Liabilities and Owner's Equity
Short-Term Asset	Short-Term Liabilities
Cash-------------------------------$19,050	Current Bank Loan---------$20,000
Money Market Acct.----------$50,000	Long-term Bank Loan----$180,000
Supplies---------------------------$60,950	
Total Short-Term Assets----$130,000	Total Liabilities-------------$200,000
Long-Term Assets	Owner's Equity
Computer---------------------- $45,000	Owner's Investment-------$120,000
Software------------------------ $45,000	
Furniture & Equipment--- $100,000	
Total Assets------------------- $320,000	Total Liabilities and Owner's Equity $320,000

The Profit and Loss Statement

Patient fees (Collected)	$550,000
General & Administration Costs	
Salaries	$110,000
Advertising	3,000
Auto Leasing	5,000
Depreciation	10,000
Insurance	8,000
Repairs & Maintenance	5,000
Dental Supplies	15,000
Taxes – Payroll	8,000
Meals	8,000
Lab Fees	50,000
Utilities	3,000
Total General & Administration Expenses	225,000
Income from Operations	225,000
Other Income (interest income)	1,000
Net Income	226,000
Proprietor's Capital (Retained Earnings), Beginning of Year	$225,000
Withdrawals (owner's income)	(210,000)
Proprietor's Capital (Retained Earnings), End of Year	241,000

The profit and loss statement can be broken down to monthly, quarterly, or yearly with percentage difference between two periods of time. This makes it easier to compare year to year or quarter to quarter.

Insurance Needed

Consideration must also be given to the many types of insurance that are necessary in a small business: malpractice, life, disability, office overhead, business/office/building, health/medical, and payroll taxes, which include but may not be limited to, depending on your location, social security, workman's compensation, and unemployment.

Malpractice is offered in two forms: occurrence and claims-made. Occurrence-based malpractice insurance provides coverage from the date the treatment was provided. Claims-made based malpractice insurance provides coverage from the date from which it was purchased and covers any malpractice claims made during that policy year. For example, with an occurrence-based policy, an endodontic procedure will be covered from the date of treatment regardless of when the malpractice claim is filed. On the other hand, a claims-made policy will cover the endodontic procedure only if the malpractice claim was filed when the policy coverage was in force, which is usually annual and renewable. The costs of an occurrence policy are higher at the beginning of one's career. Claims-made is normally less costly than the occurrence policy especially at the beginning of one's career, and then levels out after five or six years. The occurrence policy is normally always higher than the claims-made, even when the claims-made matures. If one decides to retire or change careers, the occurrence policy will continue to provide coverage while the claims-made policy will not continue coverage without the purchase of "tail coverage" to extend the claims-made policy past the annual expiration date.

Most all malpractice policies provide similar coverage. However, be aware of a waiver clause that allows the insurance company to settle a case without your consent. In other words, the insurance company may settle a lawsuit against you, even if you believe it to be a truly false claim, rather than vigorously defend the lawsuit due to the cost of defense. There are also clauses in some policies that the insurance company may recover additional costs from the dentist/defendant of a lawsuit over and above the pre-trial settlement offer. So, if the dentist does not agree to settle the case before trial per this type of clause, any amount the jury awards, above the offered settlement amount, must be paid by the dentist.

Life insurance is offered in various forms or a combination of the basic three forms of whole, term, and universal. Whole life insurance is the most expensive but allows for a cash savings for retirement while providing coverage. There are many variations, including level or adjustable premiums, though the description of these is beyond the scope of this book. Term life insurance is normally through a group. Many professional organizations, such as the American Dental Association and the Academy of General Dentistry, offer group life insurance. Group term life insurance is cheaper and provides coverage only during the term of the policy, which is normally renewable yearly. As one gets older, the costs of the policy will increase at approximately five-year increments. Universal life insurance is a combination of whole and term life insurance, which is the best of both, by allowing for maximum coverage and providing some savings with a lower premium than whole life alone. Some policies allow you to purchase more whole life or convert some of the term life coverage as the whole life is paid down. For example, the monthly premium payment for the universal life pays for both the whole life and the term life. As time passes and the whole life policy is being paid down, the monthly premium ends up paying for more whole life and less term life via the savings dividends on the whole life already purchased. It is highly advisable to purchase enough coverage to cover debts and support your family in the event of your untimely death.

Disability insurance also has its options of group and individual, and there are two types: disability/income protection and office overhead. Again, group disability policies are less costly. Disability/income protection insurance covers your income should you become disabled. There is usually a waiting period (30, 60, or 90 days) prior to the insurance providing coverage. There also may be a limitation on the amount of insurance payment depending on the extent of disability and a percentage of your actual income. Either policy should provide coverage if you are not able to do dentistry, not just any job. This is often referred to as "same occupation" coverage. Being a dentist, though a wonderful profession, is very limited in application to other job duties. If you become disabled, there are not many other jobs for which you have been trained that are as financially rewarding. Therefore, be aware of the "same occupation" clause.

Office overhead insurance is for the payment of office expenses (staff wages, utilities, rent, etc.) while you are disabled. It also has the typical waiting periods and may be adjusted accordingly as to the amount of coverage and the waiting period. It is normally significantly cheaper than disability insurance.

Cybersecurity insurance provides coverage in the case of stolen digital information that includes but is not limited to patient information and insurance information.

Sexual harassment insurance is also available to protect the dentist/owner from unintended alleged harassment claims from patients and/or staff.

With disability and office overhead, the insurer may place a waiver and not to cover a disability that is connected to a specific part of your body without an additional premium. For example, if you have a history of back problems, the insurer may place a waiver on not covering any disability due to your back for the first five years or for the entire length of the policy.

Business/office/building insurance is intended to cover losses that occur to your office or building. Depending on the policy, it should cover flooding, nondental treatment-related patient injury (slip and fall), personal property, glass breakage, fire damage, and so on. It is to protect you and your office and/or building.

The importance of health/medical insurance is obvious; to be without it could cause a devastating loss.

There are also those types of insurance required of an employer by federal and state authorities: workman's compensation, unemployment, and social security taxes.

Other regulations may be required depending on your state and local jurisdictions, which could include any or all of the following, and may not be limited to

1) Dental license
2) CPR license
3) DEA license
4) State and federal labor regulations poster
5) X-ray head certificates
6) Health department certificate
7) OSHA and bloodborne pathogens training
8) Hepatitis vaccine verification
9) IRS tax identification number
10) National Provider Identifier (NPI) number (personal and corporate)
11) HIPAA protocols.

There are three major methods of transferring a practice:

1) A phasing in, equity acquisition, or swapping equity positions from owner/seller to associate/buyer
2) A complete sale of the practice to a buyer who is outside the practice
3) A sale of the goodwill and records as a practice winds down.

Since each transition is unique, each of the methods should be modified to accommodate the parties involved. Each method has its positive and negative aspects depending on the needs of each party. Therefore, when contemplating purchasing a practice or an equity position in a larger multi-owner practice, advice must be obtained from your attorney, accountant, and practice management consultant.

Key points to remember:

1) Whether you buy or start a practice, start with a great location.
2) Seek good advice from an attorney, accountant, and practice management consultant familiar with dentistry.
3) Have a business plan ready for all possible lenders.
4) Review your insurance needs carefully.
5) Check local and state licensing and required regulations.

References

1 The New York State Small Business Development Center, *A Practical Guide to Preparing Your Business Plan* (Suffern, NY, Rockland Regional Small Business Development Center, 1992), pp. 3–5.
2 https://www.myfico.com/credit-education/whats-in-your-credit-score (accessed May 30, 2022).
3 American Dental Association, *Survey of Dental Practice, Annual Expenses of Operating a Private Practice*, 2003, p. 2.

21

Marketing for a Successful Practice

Marketing refers to the wide scope of moving goods or services from the producer (dentist) to the consumer (patient). It includes all business activity to achieve that movement, including selling, advertising, and promotion. With proper marketing, one may achieve branding of the practice to further promote the uniqueness of the practice.

Marketing has two basic forms: internal and external. Internal marketing includes all activity to promote the practice that initiates and targets those patients already within the practice with the goal to have those patients generate a referral base to your practice. It is less costly than external marketing and limited to existing patients. Be sure your practice has a good referability by having a good office appearance, presentable staff, and fair and equitable finance policies. Forms of internal marketing may include:

1) "Welcome to the practice" letters.
2) "Thank you for the referral" letters.
3) Office brochures.
4) Floss cards, toothbrushes, or other items with your name embossed on them.
5) Newsletter sent periodically (could be done via website, email addresses).
6) In office raffles for patients (gift certificates, movie or sport event tickets).
7) In Office Dental Plan.

External marketing is advertising your practice to the public. It is any notice given in a manner to attract public attention and attract new patients. It is more costly than internal marketing and therefore must be closely tracked to evaluate cost versus benefit or return on investment (ROI). It has unlimited reach but should be targeted and repetitive. Forms of external marketing may include:

1) Internet/Website/Local online information sites.
2) Television and radio ads.
3) Dental referral services as a co-op marketing.
4) Local Newspaper ads.
5) Listings in preferred provider and health maintenance organizations (PPOs and HMOs), insurance groups, or panels where the lists are available to the public.

All types of marketing should be directed to the type of patients you want. For an obvious example, you would not market an orthodontic practice in a 55-and-over community. Always keep in mind that whenever you promote your practice, whether it is internal or external marketing, the image of who you are and what your practice stands for is at stake. Your image, your practice, and your income depend on it. Poor-quality commercial advertisements only disparage your professionalism and create a poor image of dentistry as a profession (see Chapter 16).

Branding your practice is a way to show its uniqueness, such that patients will think of your practice first when in need of dental services. It is more than a logo, symbol, ad, or saying that represents your "brand." It is the sum of all promises and perceptions a practice wants its patients and prospective patients to believe about the practice's products and services such that patient motivation attaches to the psychological meaning to your logo, symbol, or saying. It is based on the perceived value to the patient. Branding strives to connect and engage with the patients on an emotional/psychological level for the patient to value being a patient of your office. Value is defined as the perceived worth in monetary units of the set of economic, functional/technical, and psychological benefits received by the customer in exchange for the price paid for a product and/ of service offering, taking into consideration available competitive offerings and prices [1]. The perceived value must be equal to or greater than the price paid. In other words, giving more in value than you get in payment. The entire staff must believe in the value of the services being offered and the cultural brand you are developing. With the multitude of advertisements on the Internet via social media and websites, it is imperative to develop a marketing strategy consistent with the value branding of your practice. It must be tied to the practice's uniqueness – the unique value of the practice as it relates to the patient. To brand a practice one must focus on the strengths of the practice and promote those strengths repeatedly over a reasonable amount of time (on average, 3–5 years), with the hope of achieving a practice brand recognition.

In 2017, Dentistry IQ did a survey on how patients choose their dentist. It was found that:

1) The dentist accepts their insurance.
2) Ease and convenience of scheduling an appointment.
3) Positive online reviews.
4) Latest technology.
5) Positive referrals from friends.

The strongest referral is that from friends and family. Some patients will forego the insurance coverage in favor of going to a dentist referred by a trusted source. It is therefore, important to develop a brand with recognition of why patients choose their dentist and support their choice through strong personal referrals.

Ethical Advertising

Advertising is relatively new to dentistry, being allowed since 1979. There have always been dentists who advertised, even in the early years of dentistry. One noted dentist advertised himself as "Painless Parker" in the early 1900s. He showed that advertising does pay: he ended his career with 30 West Coast offices, employing 70 dentists and grossing $3 million per year [2]. In the late 1970s the Supreme Court began to view professional bans on advertising as unfairly restricting competition. As a result of a recession in the late 1980s, dentists had less patients seeking care. At that time, it was called a "busyness" problem. The California Dental Association began promoting member dentists with the slogan, "We're the dentists who set the standards," to increase patients seeking care for their members. This was quickly abandoned, as it was a statement of superiority as seen by the Dental Board of California. Then, in 1999, the Supreme Court held that the Federal Trade

Commission had jurisdiction over non-profit organizations and that price advertising was allowable if it was exact, accurate, and easily verifiable. This was followed by the American Dental Association (ADA) joining with Intelligent Dental Marketing in 2007 to make professionally developed advertisements available for its members [3]. This was abandoned by 2010. So how does a dentist ethically advertise his or her practice?

The ADA Principles of Ethics and Professionalism clearly references advertising: "Although any dentist may advertise, no dentist shall advertise or solicit patients in any form of communication in a manner that is false or misleading in any material respect" [4]. It also gives advice on what constitutes "false or misleading." "With this in mind, statements shall be avoided which would:

a) Contain a material misrepresentation of fact.
b) Omit a fact necessary to make the statement considered as a whole not materially misleading.
c) Be intended to be likely to create an unjustified expectation about results the dentist can achieve.
d) Contain material, objective representation, whether express or implied, that the advertised services are superior in quality to those of other dentists, if that representation is not subject to reasonable substantiation." [5].

Unjustified expectations are easily misleading in the use of testimonials and the use of before and after treatment photos. Suggestions to avoid unjustified testimonial or portrayal include:

1) Patient should authorize in writing the use of their testimonial or portrayal.
2) Reasonable disclaimer to any statement or results achieved.
3) May use fictional situations or characters without a testimonial.
4) Fictional patient testimonials should not be permitted.

There are basically three types of advertising available to dentists in marketing their practice:

1) Comparable
2) Competitive
3) Informational.

Comparable advertising makes statements that compare one dentist to another dentist. These are usually statements of quality or superiority and are normally seen as being inconsistent with the various codes of ethics. These types of comparison advertisements may be easily misinterpreted by the public. Competitive advertising normally involves offering more products or better services at the same or lower price than that of a competitor. These are usually seen in ads with discount coupons, special prices for certain services, or even free services to entice a new prospective patient. These ads are allowed by the various codes of ethics but with great scrutiny and adherence to guidelines of the various state dental codes and statutes. Informational advertising is the most common. It contains information regarding the practice, the dentist or dentists, staff, and services available. It is generally used to inform or to educate the public on various dental topics and practice information. These types of ads are most likely to conform to the various state codes and statutes.

Before undertaking any marketing plan, be sure to review your state dental laws and codes of ethics so as to follow any necessary guidelines.

Attention must also be given to the applicable ethical principles of patient autonomy, beneficence, and veracity, as discussed in Chapter 17. These ethical principles are directly affected by dental advertising. The patient's right to self-determination must not be infringed on by misleading advertisements. Dentists, having special knowledge and having gained the public's trust through a social contract, can easily mislead a vulnerable patient and take advantage of the patient's right to self-determination with clever advertisements and marketing. To uphold the patient's autonomy, the marketing employed by the dentist should never take advantage of the patient's vulnerability [6]. It can easily mislead the patient's decision-making. A dentist should always promote benefi-cence and not promote his or her self-interest at the expense of the patient's well-being. Care should be given such that an advertisement does not shift the primary goal from patient information/education to increasing the dentist's self-interest/income.

Dentists also must be truthful in their promotion. The veracity of the advertisement should support the professionalism of dentistry. Some state statutes have placed conditions, disclosures, and disclaimers on the promotion of non-academic or non-health degrees. This includes fellow-ships earned from various dental organizations. The ADA Code of Ethics states that "some organi-zations grant fellowship status as a token of membership in the organization or some other form of voluntary association. The use of such fellowships in advertising to the general public may be misleading because of the likelihood that it will indicate to the public attainment of education or skill in the field of dentistry. Generally, unearned or non-health degrees and fellowships that des-ignate association, rather than attainment, should be limited to scientific papers and curriculum vitae" [7]. Recently, Florida courts have ruled that the Florida state statute that restricted adver-tising a general dentist's bona fide membership, credentials, and awards, such as non-specialty fellowships from non-academic organizations not recognized by the Florida Board of Dentistry, violated the Florida and US Constitutions [8]. This ruling makes way for the advertisement of earned fellowships in organizations such as the Academy of General Dentistry, the American Academy of Implant Dentistry, and the American Academy of Cosmetic Dentistry in the state of Florida. Other states are likely to follow.

Patients' vulnerability may be broken down into the type of consumer (patient) who is receiving the advertisement. There are many types of consumers. Patients may be classified into three types:

1) The skeptical patient
2) The thoughtful patient
3) The gullible patient.

The skeptical patient does not believe in anything that is self-promoted. It is very hard to get a skeptical patient to fully trust an advertisement, and thus these patients are not heavily influenced by advertisements whether or not they are false or misleading [9].

The thoughtful patient may question the information in an ad and the source from which it came. Being a reflective, questioning prospective patient, they project a "show me or prove it" atti-tude [10]. Today's highly sophisticated marketing may have a tendency to mislead a thoughtful patient, especially since the source is thought to be from a highly respected professional dentist.

The gullible patient will most likely be influenced by a misleading ad, since he or she tends to believe most advertisements, especially those from a trusted professional. The gullible patient must be protected from misleading unethical advertisements. Developing an ethical advertisement so as to not mislead a gullible patient protects all prospective patients regardless of the type of consumer he or she is. By protecting the gullible patient, our social contract is upheld and con-tinues to allow dentistry to be a profession. Hence, dentistry must maintain a wide scope in the meaning of what is misleading.

The information given in an advertisement not only formulates an image of the dentist and his or her office but also affects the patient's decision-making process. When professionals publicly compete with one another, each advertising him or herself as a better service provider than his or her peers, patients may infer that not all professionals are trustworthy, because all cannot be the best [11]. When professionals publicly compete for patients through advertising, it raises the question in the minds of the patients as to which dentist is better or more competent, when all dentists should be equally competent through licensure [6]. The patient's vulnerability should be kept paramount and the advertisement should not slide into a superiority competitiveness or even puffery, which is exaggeration concerning the quality of goods or services.

Competition for Patients

When the economy is in a recession, as was seen in the late 1970s and early 1980s, advertising becomes more competitive. Typically, when individuals offering the same professional services are located in the same community, the advertising becomes more intense and competitive. The result is that once ethical professional advertisements begin to shift toward more competitive advertising, possibly approaching puffery, this directly affects the trusting social contract that dentistry has enjoyed and brings to question dentistry's professionalism. Guarantees or warranties may begin to appear in various ads which are clearly a misrepresentation due to the fact you cannot guarantee heathcare. This also raises a legal situation of misrepresentation of the dentist's experience. If the dentist misrepresents his or her experience and the patient based his or her informed consent on that representation, then the informed consent may be found to be invalid, because the patient relied on that misrepresentation in their decision-making [12]. Therefore, if information given to the patient on which the patient did or would have relied on is found to be a misrepresentation, then the patient could sue based on an invalid informed consent. The dentist must be very careful not to exaggerate his or her experience or the results of any treatment or procedure.

With the development of practice websites, patients have easy access to any dental office's information. Websites are ungoverned and easily constructed by those not familiar with the ethical concerns of dentistry, such that the result is puffery of the dentist's true qualification. Be sure that your website designer does not use key words that may mislead potential patients, such as "cosmetic specialist." On the other hand, is it not true that the patient, now being more educated and having easy access to information, is entitled to have as much information available to enhance their decision making and choice of dentist? In fact, doesn't the patient have a right to all information regarding a dentist affecting his or her decision making? How much information is the patient entitled to, to facilitate that decision-making process and maintain patient autonomy without being misled? Does the patient influence the delivery of dental care, through his or her choices and refusals of treatment, possibly based on insurance coverage, such that the dentist's autonomy and care are directed to please the patient to the level of consumerism? These are all tough questions that need to be discussed and answered to maintain dentistry's high level of professionalism.

With the development of websites that review businesses, professionals included, and the many social media sites, dentists must be vigilant and visit these websites to check for any negative references about themselves or their practices. If a negative review or statement appears, you or someone you know should post a positive response immediately. Do not attack the reviewer. Be positive, truthful, and educative in your response. If a treatment was complained about, try to make it an opportunity to relay information relative to the benefits of the procedure, keeping the focus on the procedure and not on you.

Therefore, there are several large challenges in dental advertising. There is a need to balance the risk of lessening our professional status with the benefit of patient access to information [13]. We must maintain the professional social contract that dentistry has long enjoyed. And last, we must not become a reseller of dental appliances, dental prosthetics, or restorations.

Fee Splitting

Many specialists rely on referrals from general dentists. Those referrals must also be conducted in an ethical professional manner. There are basically four areas in which referrals may become ethically questionable:

1) Fee-splitting arrangements.
2) Referral to "the only one" to see.
3) Referral to a relation.
4) Referral within the same office.

   Most, if not all, states have statutes that do not allow fee splitting. The ADA Code of Ethics also does not allow fee splitting [14]. It is considered unethical and unlawful. Referring a patient to a colleague by telling the patient that he or she is "the only one to see" is highly suspect as being unethical. The patient's autonomy is greatly infringed on by biased information from a trusted source. Referral to a relation without revealing that a vested financial interest exists, as in spouses referring to each other, would also be suspect of being unethical. The trusting patient should be informed that the reason the referral was made primarily due to the relationship. Otherwise, the patient's best interest has then become secondary to that of the dentist's. The patient's autonomy may become compromised. The referral within the same office carries with it the same concerns as the prior two situations. The referring dentist, usually the owner, has a financial interest and obviously wants the referred patient to stay within the practice. The situation normally arises when the owner dentist refers a patient to a specialist or a general dentist ("who does all the root canals" or "who does all the extractions") and does not give the patient any other option as seen in True Case 54. The patient's autonomy and beneficence are affected by such a referral, because patients may feel obligated to stay within the practice and go to the referred-to dentist, even though it may not be in their best interest. It should be pointed out that if the referring dentist knew or should have known that the referred-to dentist is deficient in his or her patient care, the referring dentist may be held liable for the outcome of the deficient dentist's care.

True Case 54: Keeping it in the family

A patient of long standing, having a denture, came in to ask about having implants placed for a hybrid denture. The patient was given several dentists' names and accompanying referral cards by the general dentist and told to have the dentist of her choice call him. The patient had the implants placed and the hybrid made at the office of the referred-to dentist. The referring dentist saw the patient months later with the finished treatment and asked why she did not return for the fabrication of the hybrid denture. The patient responded that she was told that only the referred-to dentist's prosthodontist does the work the way he likes it and that way she would have the best result. It was later found out that the prosthodontist was the referred-to dentist's daughter-in-law working in the same office.

There are also the Federal Anti-Kickback Statute and the Stark Law that when dealing with Medicare, Medicaid, or other federal programs, it is prohibited to refer patients to a facility in which you have a financial interest.

The Logo

Before you begin marketing your practice, you should start by giving your practice a marketable image via a logo or practice name. You first need to know what kind of practice you want to be: high tech, spa dentistry, family dentistry, cosmetic dentistry, or implant dentistry, for example. In selecting a logo, take the time and do it right. You will be using it for a long time to help brand your practice. Several ways to create a logo are to seek professional help, to contact a high school or college graphic design department and hold a contest to pick the winning logo, or to simply design it yourself. The name should identify the practice and enforce the branding that you want to achieve. However, be careful not to create a name for the practice that would infer superiority, such as "Best Dental Care" or "Excellent Implants R Us." The name of the practice may identify the practice's location, such as the village, town, or area within which the practice is located (e.g., the Bellport Village Dental Group).

Besides direct external marketing, there are numerous other ways to promote your practice. Becoming directly involved in the local community is often one of the best ways to accomplish this. If you decide to follow through and join various groups, be sure to do so because you honestly care about the group and are not just in it to seek patients. A false endeavor will do more damage to your practice than not joining at all. There are many ways to become involved in your community: become active in your church, temple, or synagogue; join a community service group, such as the Kiwanis, Rotary, or Lions clubs; or participate in your children's school activities or associations. You can also take the initiative, like the dentist in True Case 55, to introduce yourself to the local hotels, bed and breakfasts, realtors, pharmacies, and merchants. Becoming a member of the local hospital staff and making yourself available for emergencies also helps to promote your practice, not just to those with emergencies, but also to the hospital staff, who will become familiar with you and may become patients.

True Case 55: Keep the patients coming

A dentist bought an existing practice in a moderately sized city. Near the location of the practice were numerous office buildings, hotels, and hospitals. The dentist took toothbrushes and business cards to the hotels for guests who may have forgotten their toothbrushes. When people visit a city, many times they are there to see someone who lives there. Not only did he receive referrals from the various places he visited, but some of the employees of the hotels became patients also. He also took business cards to the nearby pharmacies, which also resulted in new patients. He then put together welcome-to-the-area dental gift bags and gave several to the various real estate offices that handled sales and rentals in the area, to pass along to new owners and renters.

Preferred Provider Organization (PPO)

To increase the number of new patients who come into an office, some have turned to signing provider agreements with various insurance companies to be placed on a list of preferred providers. It is hoped not only that new patients will become part of the practice but also that the new managed care patient will refer others who might be self-pay patients without a reduced fee schedule, commonly referred to as collateral referrals. Dental insurance has many variations and each type has its pluses and minuses for a practice. If you become involved in any type of dental insurance as a provider, it is advised to have the patient's signature on file to process the forms and have the payment for dental care sent to the practice rather than to the patient. The following is a sample form:

> I agree to have my signature considered to be "on file" for the purposes of insurance form processing, and to be responsible for payment for any service or portion of service not covered by insurance. I authorize release of necessary information relating to the processing of dental insurance forms. I also authorize payment directly to _____.

> In order for the office to process your insurance forms more rapidly and to assist you in getting all the benefits to which you are entitled, please sign and date below.

> Signature (on file) _____ Date _____

The HMO or dental health maintenance organization (DMO) refers to insurers that pay a monthly fixed amount to the dentist per the number of assigned patient whether the patient receives treatment or not. However, when treatment is rendered, the patient pays little or no co-payment. Hence, the dentist has been paid for the treatment with the monthly capitation fee. These types of insurance plans are no longer popular.

The PPO provides its enrollees with a list of dentists who will accept a reduced set fee for any treatment rendered. There are basically three types of PPOs:

1) The agreed-upon reduced fee schedule is paid in full by the insurance company.
2) The agreed-upon reduced fee schedule is paid in part by the insurance company and in part by the patient.
3) The agreed-upon reduced fee schedule is paid in full by the patient (not a true insurance, since it is merely a reduced fee schedule available only to those patients who join the group).

Most of these types of insurance plans have some common items included in their contracts. Most include a deductible and a maximum yearly limit to benefits. They also do not pay for non-covered services, but depending on the state laws, the dentist must still abide by the reduced fee schedule even though the insurance company does not cover that service or if the yearly maximum has been reached. In other words, preferred reduced fees must be honored for those with such insurance, even beyond the agreed-upon limits and conditions by which the insurance company no longer has to pay their portion. This is called fee-capping. Many states are passing fee-capping legislation that stops insurance companies from setting fees for dental services they do not cover [15–17]. The insurance companies may also place a time limit for certain prosthodontic replacements and retreating certain dental conditions, such as scaling and root planning, within a certain number of years, regardless of the patient's need. Therefore, the need for sending preauthorizations and receiving an estimate of benefits (EOB) prior to informing patients of their coverage and co-payments is essential for proper patient communication and financial arrangements. This should be done for all crown and bridge procedures and whenever someone reviewing for the insurance company may possibly question the need for a procedure. Once the treatment plan has been finalized via a full discussion, and a proper informed consent has been obtained, the proposed treatment plan should be sent to the insurance company with complete documentation that should include periodontal charting, necessary radiographs, correct treatment codes, and a short written reason for any major treatment such as periodontal surgery, crown and bridge, and removable prosthodontics. A short narrative (one line long) on the claim form is usually sufficient to stave off rejections and usually will complete the documentation needed to expedite the claim review process. Upon receiving the EOB, the dentist may properly inform the patient of the cost of treatment, which may be a major determining factor in the patient's decision-making process. By knowing the cost of treatment, the patient may properly exercise his or her autonomy and make an informed decision.

Never guarantee what the insurance will pay, even if in receipt of an EOB as seen in True Case 56. It is only an estimate of benefit/payment. Payment is actually based on the treatment rendered, and the insurance company may change its EOB of any given procedure when the claim is reviewed for payment. Keep in mind that it is the patient's insurance, not yours.

It must be pointed out that regardless of the insurance company's acceptance or denial of proposed treatment, the liability remains with the dentist. Merely relying on the insurance company's preauthorization for treatment is not a defense if that treatment is found to be below the standard of care. Therefore, regardless of your level of involvement in various insurance plans, the risks of malpractice remain with the dentist.

There are many pitfalls when signing the insurance agreement that is given to a dentist as a "sign it the way it is or forget it" or "take it or leave it" type of contract. You do have a right to negotiate the contract, though few allow it. The ADA and its components provide contract reviews for members if they are contemplating an insurance contract. Some of the more common items of concerns are: not allowing equal time for the dentist and the insurance company to terminate the contract (a one-sided termination clause); the location for any arbitration may be in a different, distant state with different governing laws; there is no indemnification (hold-harmless clause) for the dentist if the insurance company is sued; and if the insurance company does not pay for services due to default or bankruptcy, the dentist may not seek payment from the patient. There also may be pressures put on the dentist to possibly change the manner in which he or she practices dentistry to conform to the insurance policy or benefits. Any or all of the following may be found in "preferred provider" agreements:

1) The general dentist may not perform certain covered procedures because the insurance company unilaterally decides it "is beyond the normal scope of the 'typical' practitioner" [18].
2) The dentist is pressured into treatment beyond his or her capabilities by the company, making the general dentist financially responsible for services "inappropriately" referred to a specialist [19]. The general dentist is then faced with an ethical, financial, and possibly legal dilemma.
3) The insurance company may have access to patient records for utilization reviews.

True Case 56: Insurance company approves treatment but then doesn't pay

The dentist submitted all the necessary documentation for a particular treatment for a patient. The insurance company sent back an EOB with the amount the insurance company would pay toward the patient's treatment. The patient and the dentist together developed a treatment plan and a financial agreement for the patient to receive optimum dental care to be within the EOB as much as possible. Treatment was rendered on good faith that all parties, the insurance company and the patient, would fulfill their financial responsibilities. When the insurance company received the subsequent claim, they denied payment based on review by their consultant, who determined that the treatment was not covered under the policy. Neither the dentist nor the patient was happy about the resulting situation. After many time-consuming appeals, proper payment was received.

Many states, such as New York, have prompt payment laws. Both time limits and sanctions for insurance companies are established. The insurance company has 30 days in which to dispute a claim and 45 days to pay an undisputed claim [20]. Therefore, if the claim is disputed by the patient, the insurance company is allowed a total of 75 days to pay or deny the claim. Some self-insured or self-funded programs may be exempt from these laws.

The Federal False Claims Act imposes penalties and fines on individuals and organizations that file false or fraudulent claims for payment from Medicare, Medicaid, or other federal health programs [21]. Many states also have corresponding false claims acts. There is also the Overpayment Recovery Practice Act, which requires insurance carriers to provide prior written notification within 24 months after the date that the payment was made to a health care provider when a refund is requested, or 30 months for a coordination of benefits (COB) refund [22]. Typically, dentists have 30 days to respond or the insurance carriers will automatically deduct the payment from future claims. This act applies to dentists who have contracted with the insurance company. If the dentist did not contract with the insurance company, then there are legal cases that can be cited to support the dentist not to refund the monies requested [23–25]. It is widely held that an insurance carrier is not entitled to recover an overpayment made to an innocent third-party creditor (dentist non-participating in the PPO) when:

1) that payment was made solely due to the insurer's mistake;
2) the mistake was not induced by a misrepresentation of the third-party, or
3) the third-party creditor acted in good faith without prior knowledge of the mistake [26].

More information is contained in Section 1 in "Leadership and Communication in Dentistry." Again, be sure to seek proper local legal advice regarding laws that may pertain to you and your practice.

Collections

Besides accepting payment from insurance companies, there will be patients who, even with the earnest intent, fail to pay. Patients lose jobs, lose benefits, have severe accidents, seek bankruptcy, or die. When patients' lives take a turn for the worse, be understanding. When collection is not done correctly, it may initiate an alleged malpractice lawsuit. When seeking collections of a past due balance, always preface your request by inquiring whether anything is wrong or whether there is a problem you should know about. Make several attempts to contact the patient or financially responsible party. When giving a date as to when you will call back to follow up, be sure to call back on that date. If you do not follow up as promised, then your credibility and seriousness in collecting the past due balance is threatened. Try to offer payment options to allow easier recovery of the monies owed. Additionally, charging interest, as discussed in Chapter 23, often prompts the patient to pay.

Sometimes it may be necessary to hire a collection agency. Be very sure that all treatment was well within the standard of care, all treatment protocols had been followed, and the patient's records are complete, because when a third party seeks collection, the patient may retaliate with a lawsuit (see True Case 27).

You may also seek payment through small claims court. Each jurisdiction has different limits as to how much you may sue for. Normally, the statute of limitation is the same as that of other lawsuits within the same jurisdiction or state. If the total amount you seek is above the limit, you can separate the claims according to the different completed procedures. It is advisable to wait for the statute of limitations to run its course. For example, in New York the statute of limitations is 2.5 years, so you should wait three years to go to small claims court. The statute of limitations for contract or to collect a debt is normally longer. This will lessen the possibility of the patient countersuing for alleged malpractice. However, if the patient does not have a job or any assets to allow for payment of your claim, you may be wasting your time. As mentioned previously, all treatment and records must be well within the standard of care in case the patient cross-complaints that the treatment was faulty. Sometimes accepting a very small regular payment over time is better for public relations and practice management than a more intense pursuit.

Key points to remember:

1) A good marketing plan includes internal and external marketing with eventual branding.
2) Advertising should be truthful and professionally done because it creates an image of your office and of the dental profession.
3) All marketing should be informational and should avoid statements that are misleading or make inferences to superiority.
4) Make sure to get proper advice before signing a dental insurance provider agreement.

References

1 Alice Tybout and Bobby Calder, *Kellogg on Marketing*, 2nd Edition (Hoboken, New Jersey: John Wiley and Sons, 2010), p. 188.
2 Joseph Graskemper, "Ethical Advertising in Dentistry," *Journal of the American College of Dentists*, Vol. 76, No. 1 (2009), p. 44.
3 Ibid., p. 45.
4 American Dental Association (ADA), *Principles of Ethics and the Code of Professional Conduct*, 2005, Section 5. F.
5 Ibid., Section 5.F.2.
6 Graskemper, "Ethical Advertising in Dentistry," p. 46.
7 ADA, *Principles of Ethics and the Code of Professional Conduct*, Section 5. F.3.
8 *Ducoin, DDS v. Viamonte, DDS*, Florida State Surgeon General, 2nd Circuit Court, 2009.
9 Graskemper, "Ethical Advertising in Dentistry," p. 48.
10 Ibid.
11 Jos Welie, "Is Dentistry a Profession? Part 2. The Hallmarks of Professionalism," *Journal of the Canadian Dental Association*, Vol. 70, No. 9 (November 2004), p. 600.
12 *Howard v. UMDNJ*, 172 **NJ** 537, 800 A2nd 73 (2002).
13 Graskemper, "Ethical Advertising in Dentistry," p. 49.
14 ADA, *Principles of Ethics and the Code of Professional Conduct*, Section 4.E.
15 Academy of General Dentistry, "Introducing Legislation to Prohibit Fee Capping for Non-covered Services," *AGD Advocacy Tool Kit* (December 2009).
16 Rhode Island Health care Accessibility and Quality Assurance Act, Section 1, Chapter 23–17.13.
17 Iowa State House File 2229, an Act Prohibiting the Imposition by a Dental Plan of Fee Schedules for the Provision of Dental Services that are Not Covered by the Plan. New Section 514C.3B (2010).
18 Consultants Guidelines, Criteria for Reimbursement of Specialty Referrals, Blue Cross/Blue Shield, 2010.
19 Consultant Guidelines, Inappropriate Referrals, Aetna Advantage Plus Dental/DMO, 2010.
20 NYS Insurance Code, Section 3224-a.

21 Federal False Claims Act: FCA Statute, 31 USC 3729–3733.

22 NYS Insurance Code, Section 6189.

23 *St. Mary's Med Ctr. v. United Farm Bureau* 624 NE 2nd 939, Ind. App. 1 Dist. (1993).

24 *New York Life Insurance Co. v. Guttenplan*, 30 NYS 2nd 430.

25 *Prudential Insurance Co. of America v. Couch*, 376 SE 2nd 104, W Va. Sup Ct. Of App. 1988.

26 New York State Dental Association, "Model Letter," *New York State Dental Journal*, Vol. 87, (December 2001), p. 8.

22

Social Media

Social media has become highly used by patients, dentists, and their office staff. It is a quick and easy format of communication. However, there is a need to understand the impact on our professional standing. First and foremost, when using social media to communicate with patients and/or prospective patients regarding their dental health needs or concerns, a Cyber Doctor–Patient Relationship is formed if the information given could be reasonably relied upon as a doctor to patient opinion. It is easily done through the many social media sites available (Facebook, Twitter, You Tube, Instagram, to name a few). Once the information given there is no control over its dissemination.

There are also the review sites such as Yelp, Healthgrades, and Market Circle that you have no control over in their posting reviews and or ratings. When you click on these sites for you and/or your practice, it may ask if you own this business. Be sure to claim it so no one else does. That gives you some control over the posting of information regarding you and your practice. And allows you to update as needed.

Many studies have been made regarding the impact of online reviews. In February 2012, Dental Economics found that 72% of consumers surveyed trust online reviews as much as personal recommendations and that 52% state that a positive review make them more likely to use that business. Healthgrades, in 2016 pointed out that patients are three times more likely to make an appointment when ratings and reviews are available and 74 % will change their mind based on a bad review.

Dentists also highly use websites and social media to promote their practices.
95% of dentists rely on word-of-mouth referrals,
72% rely on websites,
54% rely on social media to promote their practices,
43% use an online marketing provider,
84% manage their website/marketing on line by themselves or staff.[1].

Types and Characterizations of Social Media

There are many types of digital communication. The three basic forms are Broadcast, Relationship, and Transactional. Examples of broadcast are one-way transmissions such as blogs, advertising and online journals. Relationship broadcast is a two-way communication that aims to build the relationship as seen on Facebook, Twitter, LinkedIn, and others such sites. Transactional broadcast is the

Professional Responsibility in Dentistry: A Practical Guide to Law and Ethics, Second Edition. Joseph P. Graskemper.
© 2023 John Wiley & Sons, Inc. Published 2023 by John Wiley & Sons, Inc.

sharing of financial and personal information such as a patient filling out their health history online. All of these manners of communicating online can be seen as an endeavor to have as many opportunities for the dental office and the patient to make contact with the ease of being online. There is an avalanche of online services and products that inundate prospective patients. Therefore, the dental practice should make as many touch points with the patient as possible. This includes other forms of marketing such as local newspapers, online community information groups, support of the various local charitable organizations, and radio and television.

There are many characterizations of social media that are easily understood:

1) It has rapid, almost instantaneous distribution.
2) It can be done with little or no cost.
3) There is no limit on the longevity of the content.
4) There is a potential for anonymity and aliases.
5) Increased security difficulties.
6) It is inexpensive to create and produce the online content.
7) Allows short messages, visual content and interaction.
8) Participation can be fragments.
9) Far reaching regardless of time and place of communication.
10) Easy and cheap to duplicate and forward.
11) Potential of misrepresentation and unintended use by others.
12) Potential for sharing content out of context [2].

You Posted It, You Own It

Due to the impact on you and your practice you must maintain a professional level of any material when posting or presenting any information on social media. Do not make it your personal site. To maintain a professional level, it should be about the professional you, your staff and practice. Besides dental procedures or services offered, posting non-profit organizations, hobbies, or adventures you or staff are involved in can easily connect with patients and prospective patients. Once started it must be kept up-to-date which takes some time on a regular basis so the material posted does not get stale. This can be achieved by setting up an editorial calendar with a trusted staff member who has great communication skills and posting allowed only after your personal review.

With reviews of the practice on the various site (Yelp, Marketplace, Google Review, Etc.), an occasional negative review of less than "5" will occur. The easiest solution is "Solution to Pollution is Dilution," having more positive reviews posted. You can pursue a negative review legally based on defamation, but it is extremely hard. There are basic defenses to defamation:

The statement was based on an opinion.
The statement was true.
The statement was made regarding a public figure.

The Communications Decency Act in 1996 bars suing any website or internet provider for items posted by a third party regardless of how inaccurate or defamatory the posting is. This may be changing legislatively, but the costs can be extremely high as seen in True Case 57. Your jurisdiction may also have an "anti-SLAPP" law like California which protects defendants from defamation lawsuits that are filed to punish, deter, or silence public debate on topics of public interest, which includes health care. It also allows the court to impose attorney fees and court costs to the loser.

True Case 57: Can't stop you from posting it

A California dentist sued Yelp.com and a patient for posting a negative review. After winning, then losing on an appeal, the dentist had to pay over $80,000.00 to cover Yelp.com's attorney fees and court costs.

True Case 58: Oh yes I can stop you from posting it

A New York dentist sued several patients for defamation requesting damages of $50,000.00 to $100,000.00. Upon receiving notice of the lawsuit, the patients then either removed the posting or settled out of court.

With the discovery of a bad review, you need to be proactive, like the dentist in True Case 58, and take control and defend your "webutation" [3] You should review the various review websites, some of which have weekly reports available, on a regular basis to see if there are negative postings. Google yourself. To immediately jump in and post something in your defense is not a good idea. Each time a posting gets any following with another post regarding its content, that original post moves up the ladder in the many search sites. Hence, more attention will be brought to that original negative posting. First and foremost, dilute the negative post with many positive posts not mentioning any content of the negative post. Then, if possible, you can reach out directly to the person who posted it to privatize the situation, have them come to office to discuss it, try to remedy the situation that caused the bad post, and ask them to remove it. You can also petition the site to remove it. Of course, if it was posted by an anonymous unrecognizable name, it becomes extremely harder.

Before answering the post, stay calm and take some time to cool down, think of a positive response if you think it is necessary. Self-reflect and decide if there was any truth to the posting. A little criticism is an important part of self-improvement which goes hand-in-hand with professionalism and leadership. Maybe it is best to just ignore it. If you chose to respond, do not let an employee do it. Per HIPAA, do not address the patient's problem directly. Try to contact the patient by phone and attempt to have the patient come to the office to further discuss it. If you choose to, post that you appreciate their input, you take patient feedback very seriously, you do care about your patients, and bring attention to the procedure and its benefits. If possible, you can resolve the problem by simply redoing the treatment. I have found the best way to hopefully resolve the problem is say, "What can I do to make you happy?" If the patient requests the return of a fee, you can circumvent NPDB requirement of a written request by directly calling the patient and return the fee with a release of all claims that includes an anti-defamation clause with the understanding that he or she will remove the post.

Is It Working?

With all the investment of time and money to engage patients and prospective patients on social media, how do you know if it is working? Google Analytics and Yahoo Alerts are good places to start. Every month you can get:

Information on the number of hits on your website.
Who demographically is clicking on your website.
What pages they view and for how long they viewed it.

By following the reports, you can see if traffic to your website is increasing, at a plateau or decreasing. Demographically, you need to know if the website viewer is in your area or from some other area. There is also a bounce rate that refers to those who click on the website and leave immediately. If the number is high, over 60%, then your website is not holding the prospective patient's interest or they did not find what they were looking for [4]. The average time for someone to remain on the website is about 2–3 minutes, but may be shorter once the sought after information has been found.

When social media, including e-newsletters and e-notification for appointments, is properly used, it enhances patient communication and practice productivity. Not all patients will want to be engaged through social media, including electronic notification of appointments and maintenance visits. Be sure to ask patients as to their preference of contacting them. Some will prefer regular mail or a phone call. Through social media, contact with the patient, you can also personalize the patient contact by sending, birthday wishes, holiday wishes, "Welcome to the practice" information, and e-newsletters. If you are using a patient notification service be aware of the Telephone Consumer Protection Act of 1991 which places limitations on telephone (calls and messaging) solicitations sent with the intent of encouraging the purchase of goods and services. If violated, penalties of $1500.00 per call and/or text may be sought. The patient must have given consent for pre-recorded calls/texts and have an automatic "opt-out" feature, with reasonable accommodation to have communication by another means. It is important to have correct contact information regarding the actual telephone number or email of a patient so as not to mistakenly infringe on a non-patient with unwanted phone calls/messaging as seen in True Case 7.

So, before you post anything on social media or any electronic communication for patients or prospective patients be sure to **THINK**:

T – Is it True?
H – Is it Helpful?
I – Is it Inspiring?
N – Is it Necessary?
K – Is it Kind?

References

1 "Dental Practice Marketing Pulse Report," Prosites/Practice MOJO, 2018 Edition. (accessed and downloaded, June 5, 2022).

2 David Chambers, "Social Media Characteristics," *Journal of College of Dentist*, Vol. 79, No. 4, 2012, p. 20.

3 Chester Gary, "American College of Legal Medicine Conference presentation," (February 2018).

4 ADA Business Resources, "Is your internet marketing effective?" August 2014, Vol 45., No. 15, p. 16

23

Co-diagnosing and Gaining the Patient's Trust

The initial patient contact is made prior to the patient entering the dental office. Some patients have already made up their minds even before meeting the dentist. There are three major contacts with the patient prior to meeting the dentist. I call this the "three strikes and you're out" rule. The first hit or strike can occur when the patient sees your advertisement, website or calls your office by way of a referral. As mentioned in Chapter 21, the patient creates a mental image of you and your office based on your marketing or the way he or she is greeted on the phone. By answering "dental office," the patient is left to think whether he or she has called the right place. Proper professional etiquette must be used when answering the phone, such as, "Good morning, Dr. Smith's office, Susan speaking. How may I help you?"

The second hit or strike can occur when the patient enters the office and is greeted in person. The atmosphere of the reception area and how the patient is greeted by the staff weighs heavily on the patient's image of you and your office. It is not very welcoming to the patient to be told, "Sign in and we'll call you when it's time." The patient should be immediately acknowledged by name when he or she first comes into the office. The patient should feel truly welcome there. The reception area must be clean and up-to-date. Offering a beverage or just water is a nice welcoming gesture.

The third hit or strike can occur when the assistant or hygienist greets and escorts the patient to the operatory. As a general rule, staff should always address patients by the proper title and last name if the patient appears to be older than the staff member or over 21 years old. It is a sad situation when a 19-year-old assistant goes to the reception area and calls out "Mary" only to find out that Mary is 86 years old. If the office is rather large and the staff does not have personal knowledge of the patients, a photo may be taken on the initial visit and attached to the chart. This will prevent patient mix-up.

Depending on the people you hire, you could have three strikes against you before you or three hits in your favor before you even meet the patient.

Types of Patients

Some have referred to the presentation of a treatment plan to a patient as "selling dentistry" or "closing the sale." You cannot sell dentistry. What you are selling is yourself. You want the patient to "buy" into a trusting relationship. There are many types of patients that can basically put into three types:

Professional Responsibility in Dentistry: A Practical Guide to Law and Ethics, Second Edition. Joseph P. Graskemper.
© 2023 John Wiley & Sons, Inc. Published 2023 by John Wiley & Sons, Inc.

The Excellent Patient that easily understands the needs, value of the care needed, and follows through with the proposed treatment plan.

The Cautioned Patient that has a lot of questions, is not sure of the value of the proposed treatment, and will require a little more time to educate to relieve any doubts of the proposed treatment and it value.

The Phobic Patient that may be very talkative, cries, or needs lots of breaks during treatment requires a lot of time and staff patience in achieving a trusting doctor–patient relationship.

Hence, you are selling trust. However, trust cannot be sold; it must be developed, nurtured, massaged, and earned. Therefore, every contact you or your office has directly or indirectly with a current or prospective patient must honor that ever-developing trust. For more information on patient interaction see Section 2 "Leadership and Communication in Dentistry."

Making the Appointment

After the initial contact, an appointment must be made. Be sure to leave enough time to educate the patient, to allow any questions, and to gain the patient's trust. Focus on the patient and take some interest in his or her hobbies, job, and/or family. People love to talk about themselves. Try to "connect" with the patient by finding some common interest. Many times it may be a staff member who connects with the patient through some common interest or similar family situation. Being on time and being organized also helps to build that trust. If your patient chart is haphazard, disorganized, incomplete, or you do not know how the software works, the patient may feel the same about their quality of care. When discussing needed treatment, always keep in mind that patients typically will be using discretionary income, unless it is a more urgent health situation such as in the case of pain or swelling. Being rushed, fumbling through a chart, or not being able to properly use the software, does not help develop the patient's interest to turn dental needs into dental wants.

Always keep the focus on how the treatment will benefit the patient and the value the treatment has to the patient. Many dentists spend too much time discussing how something will be done, or how good the dentist is, rather than the benefit to the patient. To understand the patient's wants, ask open-ended questions that require more than a simple "yes" or "no." For example, "How may I help you?" "What are your concerns about your teeth?" "What do you like or not like about your teeth?" "Are there any questions concerning your dental health you would like to ask?" Then give the patient time to formulate and answer or ask a question. In today's production and goal-oriented practice, the dentist is often too hurried and does not focus on the patient as a person. Take the time to involve and educate the patient, raising his or her "dental IQ" up a notch. Just raising the patient's "dental IQ" or awareness slightly by involving the patient allows him or her a better understanding and appreciation for dentistry; and, creates a dental want rather than just fulfillment of a dental need. You must motivate the patient.

Patient Motivation

Motivation entails three parts: a goal, knowledge, and attitude which together give value to the dental services offered. The patient must be given a goal that is attainable. A patient will not be motivated by a treatment plan that is financially unattainable. The patient must have understanding of the goal. A patient will not be motivated if he or she does not understand the goal and its benefit to him or her. The patient must change his or her attitude. A patient will not be motivated to accept the treatment plan even if he or she understands the attainable goal unless he or she wants to accept it. The use of digital imaging allows monitor-sized radiographs and photographs allowing patients to easily see and understand their dental needs. There are also many patient education software programs that provide a visualization of various dental needs and how treatment is provided. An intra-oral camera or a patient mirror may also be used to educate the patient about his or her needs. However, it is the patient's involvement, not just a dictation of treatment plan, that brings about a true co-diagnosis. The more patient involvement, the more the patient takes part in diagnosing or acknowledging his or her dental needs and wanting treatment. To help you stay focused on the patient, be attentive to body language and keep eye contact. Good listening not only brings the patient into a co-diagnosis, but helps you in your understanding and care for the patient. Some patients need more than just one appointment to understand their dental needs, so be available for another appointment, if needed, to answer any further questions the patient may have. Also be aware that many patients have different beliefs regarding the importance of dental care due to direct family beliefs or cultural/social beliefs. From patients with personal beliefs that everyone ends up with a denture by the time they are 40, as seen in True Case 59, to patients with social/cultural beliefs that betel nut/leaf and areca nut chewing is healthy, these ideas play a large part in a patient's preconceived understanding of dental care. By taking the time to ask questions to understand the origin of the patient's beliefs and habits, you will build trust and properly educate the patient to accept needed dental care by their involvement in a co-diagnosis. As the saying goes, "Sharing is caring." More information on patient motivation can be found in Chapters 7 and 8 in "Leadership and Communication in Dentistry."

True Case 59: Denture time

A mother brought her 21-year-old daughter to see the dentist due to pain. The mother (before the Health Insurance Portability and Accountability Act [HIPAA]) explained to the dentist that everyone in the family usually gets their dentures by the time they are 25, and, her daughter being 21, it was now the daughter's time to get a denture. Additionally, the cost of ideal dental treatment was well beyond the family's financial abilities. The daughter, having several missing teeth and several that were severely carious, agreed with the mother. The dentist discussed the importance of trying to keep a few teeth for retention of a partial denture and/or to reduce the amount of ridge resorption that will take place over time if a denture were made. The dentist relieved the pain and had the daughter back to discuss some options to save some teeth, at a cost no more than that of a denture. By taking the time to listen and communicate with the patient, and the mother in this case, the dentist was able to raise the patient's dental understanding and provide a great service for the daughter.

Co-diagnosing With the Patient

Co-diagnosing is not just diagnosing and then having a discussion lead by the dentist. It starts with the building of a trusting doctor–patient relationship. It is not about what is to be done but rather what condition the patient is in and how treatment will benefit them. Thus, bringing the value to the proposed treatment to the patient's attention. This has been referred to as Valued-Based or Backward Diagnosing: Starting with the benefit of the treatment rather than the treatment itself thereby giving value and a reason for the patient to proceed.

With the development of the Internet giving easy access to information, most patients are some-what aware of dentistry, the importance of dental health as it relates to total health, and the various treatments available per "Dr. Google." They have become Internet educated. Hence, you must make yourself aware of how to substantiate or redirect the patient's understanding that was sought on the Internet. Some patients will actually ask for a specific treatment that may not be in the proper sequence to achieve the goal the patient ascertained from the Internet. You must be able to redirect the patient so you do not become an agent of the patient doing only what they think should be done or only what insurance will pay for. You need to become an advocate of the patient to redirect and achieve proper dental care.

Once the treatment plan has been mutually accepted, the next step the patient must take is the payment for the treatment. There are many ways to finance treatment when the patient cannot afford the full treatment fee: insurance co-payment (as discussed in Chapter 21), outside financing such as CareCredit or Citi Patient Finance, credit cards (Visa, MasterCard, American Express, Discover), debit cards, or a signed financial agreement.

You may also choose to deduct a percentage (5%–10%) of the total fee or to spread out the treatment over time to make it more affordable (phasing the treatment over one or two years) to help the patient receive the dental care needed. If so, you must still fulfill all the requirements of financing.

Outside sources of patient financing, such as CareCredit, Citi Patient, or Chase Health Advance financing, normally do not charge interest to the patient for 3 to 18 months, depending on the agreement. The outside creditor then pays the full amount of the treatment plan less a set percentage to the dentist even before treatment has begun. If you decide to finance the treatment within your office, you must fulfill the Truth in Lending Act. Always try to keep internal financing to no more than three months, due to the fact that the patient's life may take a different turn than expected, such as loss of job, divorce, move away to relocate, or severe injury. To eliminate some problems, it is advised to have the patient pay at least half of any treatment that involves lab fees at the start of treatment. In that way, at least the lab bill would be a covered expense. All financing should be discussed with a designated staff member who has a good understanding of dental insurance and the costs of providing quality dentistry. Many times when the dentist gets involved in the finances, patients often plead for a "break" on the costs. The dentist, wanting to be the "good guy," will play into this bargaining or negotiation for the lowest price. There is also the situation when the patient informs the receptionist that the dentist said it would cost less than what the receptionist is now asking for; when, in fact, the dentist properly informed the patient of the cost. To prevent such practice management and public relations problems, it is best to refer all financing inquiries to a staff member with proper financing knowledge. Therefore, it will not turn into a "who said what" problem.

The federal truth-in-lending disclosure statement for professional services rendered requires specific information. Even if you choose not to charge interest, you must still have a disclosure statement per the Truth in Lending Act and Regulation Z. As with any legal agreement, proper legal advice is necessary [1]. The disclosure statement must have the following:

1) Patient's name.
2) Payer's name, if different from the patient's.
3) Full fee for services.
4) Amount the payer owes.
5) Any down payment (half of the total if involving dental labs).
6) Remaining amount being financed or loaned.

7) Number of installments.
8) Amount of each payment.
9) When each payment is due.
10) Date when contract is to be paid in full.
11) Costs incurred if the amount financed is not paid in a timely manner (and any service charges or interest if applicable).
12) Signature and date and a copy to the payer.

Be aware that the requirements needed to finance treatment internally may change as new government regulations evolve.

After all the effort to involve the patient in his or her treatment, most patients judge dentists by everything but the actual quality of their care. Patients judge dentists by some of the following criteria:

1) Painless injection.
2) Painless treatment, including that of the hygienist and staff.
3) On-time, well-run office.
4) Whether all questions (even dumb ones) were addressed, and how they were addressed.
5) Prompt emergency service.
6) Office up to date in technology and decor.
7) Help with insurance company paperwork.
8) Convenient location and hours.
9) Office cleanliness.
10) Appearance of doctor and staff.

Key points to remember:

1) People normally do not sue people they like and trust, so you should build trust at all times.
2) Communication and patient involvement in co-diagnosis is the key to building patient trust.
3) Do not become a lender of money such that you create financial issues that could cloud the patient's view of treatment quality.
4) Communication and trust are keys to good risk management.

Reference

1 The Truth in Lending Act (TILA), Title I of the Consumer Credit Protection Act.

24

Employee Management

Employees have been previously discussed in the sections on statutes in Chapter 2 and general basic employment concepts in Chapter 15. However, there is still another area of employee management that may affect the new dentist even more: hiring, firing, and rewarding employees.

Always attempt to have the best employees, who complement your personality and the way you practice. If you are a quiet and reserved type, you would not want all your employees to also be quiet and reserved. A team takes many different types to be successful. After buying a practice and retaining the employees or starting a new practice, the need to hire will arise. Start with a well-written ad with a full description of the type of employee you want. "Dental assistant needed (call this number)" will not attract the best applicants. For example, "Dental assistant needed full-time in Jones Village. Must be energetic, have initiative, and 2-year minimum experience to join growing dental team (call this number)" is a better approach and will attract the more qualified applicants. Other places to look for a new employee are the local dental society, local dental assisting school, employment websites, or temporary help agencies. Temp agencies and on-line employment services charge a fee for placing an applicant with you. However, there are also costs to placing an ad in the newspaper or on a website.

Once the applicant comes for an interview, besides following all the recommendations in Chapters 2 and 15, you will need to decide if this is the best applicant for the job. Always ask open-ended questions that require more than a yes or no answer to observe the potential employee's speaking abilities. Let the applicant talk. Many times applicants will talk themselves into or out of a job. References should be asked for and followed up. When calling a former employer, listen to what is *not* being said. The reference should be very positive and highly recommending the applicant. If it is not, then be attentive. The foremost question to ask is if they would rehire the applicant again. Have the applicant write a short sentence or two, in order to observe his or her spelling and handwriting, especially if hiring a receptionist. Regardless of the job position, all applicants should be told everything that is expected of them and all practice policies. Employees become disgruntled when the job they accept is not the job they interviewed for and expected.

Those applicants who are being seriously considered may be given a working interview. In a working interview, the existing staff (including the dentist) may then have a chance to evaluate a new potential member of the team. It is like an informal group interview. Do personalities clash or do they enhance the practice? It is normal for applicants to overstate their competency like the applicant in True Case 60 in their desire to get a job, attempting to appear to be the best applicant; their true abilities will show only after being hired.

Professional Responsibility in Dentistry: A Practical Guide to Law and Ethics, Second Edition. Joseph P. Graskemper.
© 2023 John Wiley & Sons, Inc. Published 2023 by John Wiley & Sons, Inc.

True Case 60: Please believe me

A small office was seeking to hire a receptionist who could also step in as a dental assistant when needed. The applicant put down on her resume that she also assisted before becoming a receptionist in another office. When the dentist noticed she also assisted, the dentist thought of hiring her. When the applicant was asked how long she assisted she stated "I only observed dental assisting when I was in a dental assistant school." Upon further questions, it turned out that the previous office she assisted in was not a dental office. Needless to say, she was not hired.

On the other hand, be aware that a one-day working interview where everything is in a different place and staff–patient interaction is not what the applicant is used to may make it a little harder to adjust than the applicant thought.

Several times throughout your career as an owner/dentist, you will have to hire someone during a staffing shortage who doesn't know dentistry. When the economic environment stresses the pool of applicant, you must be willing to train. Hire the person with the personality and the attitude you believe you can work with. During the 90-day try-out period, observe if the new hiree's personality and attitude makes up for the lack of dental knowledge through their want to learn and work with the rest of the staff: someone who picks up on the office culture and wants to be "In".

Testing the Waters

As mentioned in Chapter 15, a 90-day trial period is highly recommended to "test the waters" for all: the dentist, the staff, and the new employee. During this time remember that the new employee should be attempting to become one of the team, and not just showing up for a job. During this time, see if the employee fulfills the "5 Cs":

1) Confident: Does the applicant appear confident in his or her job duties? Does the applicant take initiative or make an effort to take on the job? Must he or she be told to do every little step? The more experienced the applicant is, the more initiative is expected.
2) Comforting: Does the applicant show empathy and not just sympathy? Is he or she a good listener for the patient?
3) Caring: Does the applicant show understanding of the patient's situation, the office protocol, and the treatment provided?
4) Competent: Does the applicant show a high level of knowledge as per his or her stated experience?
5) Cleanliness: Does the applicant know what clean means? Is his or her personal hygiene acceptable? In the health care field, you and your practice will be judged on the cleanliness of your office and the appearance of your staff.

Office Culture Integration

The next step to the possible integration of the new applicant is to examine his or her personality compatibility. Some have suggested personality tests, which may be offensive to some and somewhat costly to administer. Some have suggested that one should always strive to seek the best in the applicant pool. However, a situation where everyone has a strong personality and wants to be in power makes for a very competitive work environment; intra-staff competition may hinder the team building you are trying to achieve. Everyone can't be office manager. The best way to develop a team that will work together for the betterment of the whole office is to have a composite of personalities. For fun, I have divided up various office personalities by type as they relate to five animal traits: bear, owl, rabbit, deer, and monkey.

The bear is that type of person who, when given a job with a goal, will stick with it no matter what. This type of person is strong-minded and hard-working. This trait can easily be seen in most office managers or someone who would be good working with accounts receivables/collections from patients and insurance companies.

The owl is that type of person who will ponder most job duties prior to their undertaking. This type of person is contemplative and thoughtful and may question things more than the others. He or she tends to be a better listener and often has thoughtful input into the dynamics of the office. After thinking about the situation, this type of person often comes up with great suggestions for the practice.

The rabbit is that type of person who is able to go from one job duty to another without skipping a beat, simply "hopping" from one situation to another successfully. This type of person does best in a busy office and when given multiple job duties. A good quality for the main receptionist or main assistant.

The deer is that type of person who works quietly without drawing attention to him- or herself. When attention is given to this person, he or she will simply stop as if staring into headlights. This type of person does best with routine job duties that require continuous attention, such as calling or confirming maintenance visits and reactivation of patients who haven't been in for a couple of years.

The monkey is that type of person who is very talkative and always looking at the fun side of the situation. He or she is the first one to crack a smile or to make someone smile. This type of person is needed in every office to relieve stress; after all, "Humor is the shock absorber of life." The light-hearted approach of this type of person bonds the team together.

No one person has only one trait nor does a composite give equal weight to each of the traits. Most staff will have a few of the above traits, with some traits being more dominant than others. The secret to a successful team is to have the right combination to allow individuality and a cohesiveness. As with any team, there will be days when the team is "on" and other days when the team is not. It is hoped that this interaction of the staff's different personalities and qualities becomes synergistic so "off" days are easily overcome and is noticed by patients as a reflection of a caring team of professionals. If the interaction is negative, that will also be noticed by patients. Hence, it is important to get the staff combination right. It may take several attempts to find the right person for the right job.

However, to attract the right team and maintain them, you need a person to be the team leader: the dentist. To be the team leader you must wear several "hats" at the same time: player, coach, manager, and owner:

PLAYER: Working together with your employees.
COACH: Bringing the best out of each team member and cheering them on.
MANAGER: Keeping a great team together and motivated.
OWNER: Making sure there is a profit.

So, at times you must be a friend and co-worker, a supervisor, a problem solver, and a decision maker. Thus, the most important questions for you to answer when hiring someone are: Is he or she good for the practice? Can I work with him or her? Can he or she work with the rest of the staff? You or the rest of the dental team should not have to change to accommodate a new employee. Remember, you are trying to get the right people in the office canoe in the right seats, facing the right way and paddling in the right direction!

The Paperwork

Once the employee is hired and given an employee manual (see Chapter 10 in "Leadership and Communication in Dentistry"), be sure all forms are filled out and/or filed, including but not limited to:

1) W-9.
2) I-9.
3) State-mandated Workman's Compensation Insurance.
4) State-mandated Unemployment Insurance.
5) Other tax forms.
6) OSHA and blood-borne pathogens training.
7) Heptavax given or signed by physician.
8) Employment "at will" contract, if state law allows.
9) Wage Theft Prevention Form (at time of hire and yearly by February 1).

The owner dentist carries the ultimate responsibility to make sure all employment forms are up to date, proper infection control guideleines are followed, and there is proper training of the staff for OSHA, blood-bourne pathogens and HIPAA, to name a few.

True Case 61: Dr. Chadwick v. Board of Registration in Dentistry (MASS)

Dr. Chadwick relied heavily on his staff to properly follow the many rules and regulations regarding infection control, OHSA, CDC, and HIPAA guidelines. Upon discovery that he and staff were disposing used aneasthetic carpules in the regular trash, investigation was started into his practice regarding infection control and other rules and regulations. It was found that he failed:

To provide proper training.
To maintain records on Heptavax vaccinations.
To complete his own declination to be Heptavax vaccinated.
To have monthly meetings per the OSHA and CDC guildelines.
To have an exposure control plan.
To conduct weekly autoclave spore testing.
To properly dispose of glass carpules.
To properly dispose of blood-soaked cotton balls and gauze.

A good risk-management tool, if you are still using paper treatment notes, is to have all employees upon hire give a sample of their signature and initials. It may become useful in the event of a law suit and questions that arise as to who wrote what in the chart. Likewise, all newly hired employees should have their own password when using computerized charts to allow for possible future audits.

Evaluation and Appreciation

Evaluation of the employee is essential to creating a great dental team wherein there is mutual professional respect for everyone on the team as well as for the patients. Evaluation should start during the 90-day trial period. To help a new employee adjust to the new office, the employee should be met at the end of each day to discuss how the day went. This is not a time to berate or reprimand the new employee but to help him or her in job duties, to provide encouragement, and to help him or her become a team member. The new employee should be informed of what to improve on, as well as encouraged in the things done right. A new employee is typically eager to do a good job and be accepted as part of the dental team. Time should be spent on how to improve the new employee's performance and not just on what they did wrong. Positive re-enforcement has a better return than negative fault finding. When meeting with any employee or the entire office, the "sandwich" approach works rather well. This approach begins with mentioning and giving credit for the good things that have happened. The middle should mention the things that need improvement. It should not be a harsh criticism of what's wrong, but what needs to be corrected to make the practice better. The end should summerize that which was mentioned to be improved upon and how it will be undertaken to allow the practice to meet its potential and be the best it can be. It is important to give all three areas approximately equal time, and to allow the employee staff to respond, have input or to discuss any issues he/she/staff may have. As with all meetings with employees, be sure to make written notes in the employee's chart. As mentioned before, a witness should be present if the meeting is regarding a serious problem, such as firing.

When evaluating front-office personnel, it should be understood that they are the gatekeepers of the practice. They control the patients coming into and going from the practice. They are usually the first and last encounter during the patient's dental visit. Hence, evaluation should center around those most important parameters. Some of the inquires could be: Do they keep track of cancellations/no shows? Do they follow up on missed appointments? Are patients being properly scheduled, including maintenance visits? Are financial arrangements and collections acceptable? Does everyone get along and work together?

The back office staff is a true complement to the dentist in providing dental care. Patients often feel more comfortable asking questions of the staff regarding treatment rather than the dentist. Therefore, the staff must not only be knowledgeable but also able to put the patient at ease when discussing the treatment. Hence, the evaluation could include inquires such as: Are all the assistant's or hygienist's job duties fulfilled, including cleanliness? Does the employee make the patient feel comfortable enough to ask questions, and he or she give acceptable answers? Does the employee have empathy for those patients in need? Does everyone get along and work together?

Many offices have an annual personalized employee evaluation. The larger the office, the more important it is to have such annual meetings with each employee individually to maintain connection with that employee. Be very congnisent that the employee attaches an annual raise with such evaluation. It should be pointed out to the employee that such an individual meeting is not about raises, though if you choose to give a raise is up to you. I have found after employing numerous staff for many years, some over 20 years, an annual raise is very hard to maintain, because over time the pay exceeds the job. Instead. there are two ways, besides giving more benefits, to show appreciating in the paycheck. Whatever raise you were going to give, for example, 50 cents/hour, add up the hours normally worked for the year and round down to a number which may work out to $4–500.00 and make a lump payment or payment over a couple of pay periods to show appreciation. This will work for awhile, but ends the yearly building up of the base wage which increases annually with each yearly wage increase. Another way is to have a bonus system whereby when the office does well, the employees get a bonus. This eliminates the toll on overhead when there are a couple of slower months. The bonus should be easy to reach and based on collections. Once the threshold amount (that which you need to cover all expenses including your paycheck for a normal month) is collected, a $50.00 to a $100.00 bonus is given with adding small increments going past the threshold to act as an incentive.

It has been found that wages or salaries are not the number one reason for an employee to be happy with his or her job.

What Employees Want	What Employers Think Employees Want
1. Interesting work	5
2. Appreciation of work	8
3. Feeling "in on things"	10
4. Job security	2
5. Good wages	1
6. Promotion/growth	3
7. Good working conditions	4
8. Personal loyalty	6
9. Tactful discipline	7
10. Sympathetic help with problems	9 [1]

To keep employee morale up, there are many ways to "show your love." Some of the simple things you can do are:

1) Say "Thank you," and mean it, after work each day.
2) Remember their special days (birthdays, anniversaries, children's birthdays).
3) Arrange a social outing (bowling, miniature golf, "happy hour").
4) Have a "bravo board" or designate an "employee of the month."
5) Send flowers (or bagels, cake, fruit basket) to the office.
6) Hand out car wash or restaurant certificates, lottery tickets, or lunches.

Feel free to use your imagination! And don't forget the element of surprise.

Even with the best intentions, things may not run smoothly. Staff mistakes that cause disruption within the office can be many and various. Some of the more common snafus are not firing an employee for continued lateness, gossiping, or nastiness toward other co-workers. The sooner you approach the problem, the sooner it will be solved. Ignoring the problem only lets something grow and mature into a real office crisis. If it is between two individuals, it is best to have each person sit down to reconcile the problem. If not resolvable, then decisions must be made for the betterment of the whole office. Sometimes it is better to terminate an employee than wait to see if he or she will change. People usually do not change.

Problems can arise when there is no written office policy for all employees. It is wise to have employees sign that they have received that manual on the day of hire, so as to reduce any miscommunication. Giving benefits too soon leads to the employee expecting more and more as length of employment increases. Normally, no benefits should be given during the 90-day trial period, and certain goals should be met to obtain raises or other benefits as spelled out in your employee manual. And last, do not give too much power or access to any one employee. Many problems have arisen when one employee has access to the business checkbook and the employer's computer and files. It is too large of a temptation for the employee, so why take the risk? More employee management information can be found in Section 2, Part 2 in "Leadership and Communication in Dentistry."

Key points to remember:

1) Attract and hire good employees.
2) Keep all required employee records up to date.
3) Do not allow intra-office "bad attitudes" to fester.
4) Always acknowledge the employees' contribution to the dental team.

Reference

1 Jackie Bailey, "Lions and Tigers and Bears ... Oh My!" *Dental Economics* (October 2007), p. 146.

25

Multispecialty Practice

Now that you have all the elements to establish a great practice, what's next? Many dentists look to bring in an associate to expand their practice or to have a little more time for themselves. Adding an associate brings a new dynamic to the practice. The associate may be the same type of practitioner or may have a different specialty. Over a short period of time a multispecialty practice may be formed with the right team that allows complete, all-phases of dentistry to be completed in one office. It is extremely convenient if specialists are present in the same office as the general dentist which allows complete patient care during one visit, especially if the patient has to travel a far distance for treatment. But let's begin by seeing how to turn a general practice into a premier multispecialty practice where patients may come even from other countries for treatment, as they did for my former practice.

The Set Up

As the general practice grows, a wider range of treatment should be offered. Most times it begins with a periodontist and then you can add specialists as the practice is able to support each addition to the group. Along with the addition of each specialist, the staff has to become more proficient in the needs of the various specialties. This also brings new and unexpected problems that need to be addressed. With the addition of the associate–specialist, careful attention needs to be given to independent contractor status as defined by the Internal Revenue Service (IRS) (see Chapter 19).

First and foremost, the general dentist usually is the team leader in that he or she must have excellent technical, diagnostic, and communication skills. The owner dentist must be proficient in all phases of dentistry so when a specialist leaves, he or she can cover that specialty's emergency and follow up care till a new specialist is found. The owner dentist is what I call a "Super-Generalist." Then the general dentist, usually the owner in such a situation, needs to have the office space to accommodate a multispecialty practice. Also needed are the patients to fill the schedule of all the dentists involved. So how does one bring life to such an endeavor? Find the right location.

The ideal location would be on a major roadway or other area that has easy access and visibility. Trying to start a multispecialty practice while hidden on the fourth floor in a large office complex is a large hurdle to overcome. Once the location is found, the next consideration is to have enough space for growth. Having 10 chairs/operatories, as I had, may be excessive, while the minimum is six: two for hygienists, one or two for general practice, and the rest for specialists. However, if you plan on having orthodontics or a large pedodontic patient load, then a minimum of two to three

Professional Responsibility in Dentistry: A Practical Guide to Law and Ethics, Second Edition. Joseph P. Graskemper.
© 2023 John Wiley & Sons, Inc. Published 2023 by John Wiley & Sons, Inc.

chairs in an open bay is needed to accommodate the patients. One of the specialty rooms should be large enough to allow for sedation equipment and additional needed personnel for general anesthesia. The actual design to facilitate proper staff and patient flow throughout the office is beyond the scope of this section.

Now that the office is open in a great location, proper, professional, ethical marketing needs to be initiated. If you are the creative type, think of some ideas that could be marketable; write them, draw them, and take them to the venue in which you plan to promote your practice. Most magazines, newspapers, and social media promoters have a talented staff who will be able to put the finishing touches on your ad. Marketing may be needed to let prospective patients know that you exist. See Chapter 21 for more information.

As the practice grows, the first specialist to incorporate is the periodontist, because most adult patients will have a need for periodontics and/or implants. The general dentist should then refer all periodontal patients, including those with simple or moderate periodontitis, to the periodontist, to allow him/her to reach their potential as a practice asset. There should be an increase in hygiene appointments due to the need for three-month periodontal maintenance visits following scaling and root planing or periodontal surgery. If only referring the worst periodontal cases, the periodontist will not be utilized to their fullest potential and decide that he or she is not busy enough and leave.

Who's Next

The next specialist to join the group should be an orthodontist or endodontist. Again, if an orthodontist is added, be sure you have the physical layout required for him or her to make that part of the practice efficient. The endodontist will need a room large enough to accommodate an intra-oral microscope. He or she will most likely need only one room to meet the patient load. Many general dentists are fairly proficient in endodontics. However, when you add an endodontist to your practice, I highly recommend that even if you are well within your abilities to treat some endodontic cases, you should refer all endodontics to the specialist, except those procedures to alleviate pain (in which case, temporize and then refer). The endodontist's schedule will become filled more quickly and the general dentist may then be able to give more time to preferred procedures.

As the practice grows, the addition of an oral surgeon may well benefit the group. With oral surgery, certain upgrades, such as recovery area, crash cart, and general anesthesia licensure, are needed due to the fact that general anesthesia is now being used in your group practice. Check with your jurisdiction regarding special state requirements for general anesthesia. There will always be discussion of who will be doing those procedures that cross over to other specialties, such as implant placement/restoration and minor tooth movement. For continuity of treatment and a mutual practice philosophy, it is best that those crossover procedures be openly discussed and delegated to one or the other specialist, or a mutually agreed upon intra-office referral policy.

Depending on the interests of the general dentist, a prosthodontist may join the group. However, remember that patients are concerned about fees. If two dentists provide the same procedure, and one is a specialist who charges more, some patients will gravitate to the least costly. This undermines the effectiveness of having the specialist. Therefore, maintain the same fee schedules. Patients will then most likely opt to have the specialist perform the procedure, and thus he or she will be more productive. As a side note, no matter whether the general or specialist treats the patient, both will be held to the same standard of care. Referring the patients to the specialists allows you, the general dentist, to concentrate on those procedures you prefer to do and to allow the specialist to be useful and productive to the practice. In that manner the practice, the owner, the associate specialists, and your new multispecialty practice will fulfill and surpass all expected potential.

True Case 62: I want to pay more

A husband and wife came to the office for new dentures that were much needed. They wanted to come at the same time. The husband was appointed to the general dentist and the wife was appointed to the prosthodontist. Both dentists used the same lab and the same materials. The only difference was that the prosthodontist liked to set his own maxillary anterior six teeth and charged $200 more. When it came time for final payment upon delivery of the dentures, the husband questioned why his was less. In the attempt to explain that both were the same except for the prosthodontist setting the anterior six teeth, he was slightly upset that he did not get as good of a denture as his wife. After that date the owner general dentist changed all his fees to the specialist fees.

Some of the specialists who join a group practice may also have their own practices and use the office as a satellite office. Others may be working in several offices. All associate specialists should work part-time to better fulfill IRS criteria. All the specialists should be required to have a contract so there will be no misunderstanding of each party's responsibility. It is best for each specialist to provide those instruments particular to his or her specialty. This helps to fulfill the IRS criteria, as pointed out in Chapter 19. Otherwise, the owner dentist will become a dental supply house as specialists come and go, each of which often has different instrument needs to provide the same specialty procedures. Additionally, it is highly recommended that employment of specialist associates should be made directly and not simply through another specialty group or practice contracted to provide the specialist. Again, continuity and practice philosophy may differ greatly even among partners of the same practice. The composition of the practice will change every time a new specialist is added or replaced. One specialist may recommend to the patient that the tooth be saved, while the other specialist from the group may recommend that it be extracted. The patient is then confused as to whose recommendation he or she should follow. This type of situation does not occur often, but when it does, the owner dentist should meet with the patient to discuss the options and lead the patient to a proper, mutually agreed-upon treatment. When these types of situations occur, it is up to the owner to deal with them, since he or she has a better understanding of the practice's philosophy.

In addition to the typical wording in the specialist's contract, mention should be made of the noncompete/restrictive covenant, the manner of payment, and what is expected to be provided by the specialist. A complete discussion of the contractual issues is beyond the scope of this chapter. Nevertheless, some mention is necessary. Noncompete or restrictive covenants are not a major concern until a specialist associate leaves and he or she opens an office one block away, followed by all the orthodontic or periodontic patients who leave the group practice (see True Case 47).

Show Me the Money

The best manner of payment is based on collections. To base payment on production makes it very difficult for the owner dentist, because it is hard to pay the specialist on production when full payment has not been received due to numerous appointments for a procedure (this can obviously be broken down to each appointment). There is also delayed insurance payments and adjustments, patient payment plans, or credit card programs such as MasterCard, American Express, CareCredit, adjusted PPO fees and their discount rates that affect the proper payment to the specialist. There are also the high overhead procedures, such as implants and orthognathic surgeries that may require specific agreed-to splitting of those expenses. These discounts and adjustments should be made on the specialists' collections for proper remuneration. To keep all well-informed, a daysheet showing the daily treatment charges and collections for each specialist for the days they work and a monthly accounts receivable should be given to the specialist. There will be patients who see all the dentists on several appointments. In such cases, the deciding factor as to who gets paid first should be based on first in time treatment.

It is highly advisable for the specialist/associate to also maintain proper records of treatment rendered and accounts receivable. On a quarterly basis, those records should be checked/audited against the office data to ensure proper compensation. Sometimes even with current sophisticated dental software, an entry could be made in the wrong doctor's ledger and will need to be adjusted accordingly.

Another hurdle is the use of auxiliary personnel. To be most efficient, allowing the specialist to "use" one of the general dentist's assistants may be fine when starting out and the schedule is slower. However, when you randomly put a dentist and an assistant together, hoping for the best, the true potential of the specialist may not be met. Also, to help meet the IRS criteria, it is best to have the specialists either bring their own assistants or to train an existing one. If two people want to work together, there is a synergy that comes about that allows the associate specialist to meet his or her full potential within the practice. An assistant may be excellent in general dentistry; but when assisting, a periodontist or oral surgeon may faint at the sight of complex surgical procedures.

At the beginning, the reception personnel should be able to fulfill the needs of all the dentists interchangeably. However, as the new format of a multispecialty practice develops, it is best to assign certain receptionists to individual dentists/specialists. This will lead to a better understanding of the specialist's scheduling needs and the individual financial needs of the different types of patients. Whether the practice is a fee-for-service without any preferred provider or health maintenance organizations (PPOs or HMOs), or heavily involved in dental insurance, it is always good practice management to have a secure financial policy in place for the entire practice. The financial agreements for an orthodontic practice are different from those for an oral surgery or general practice. Hence, by matching up the interest of each assistant and receptionist with the appropriate specialist, the true potential of the practice is met not just in patient treatment but also in patient financing and practice profit.

Another area of concern is the referral from outside the office and those referred to specialists within the practice. It is obvious that referrals from outside the practice directly to the specialist must be referred back to the referring dentist to maintain an ethically professional relationship. However, those being referred within the practice are subject to the ethical concerns regarding the financial interests/gain of the owner (see Chapter 15). The autonomy of the patient must not be undermined by referring all patients to your specialists without giving the option to see another outside specialist. The patient must be informed of all information that a reasonable person would want to have to make an informed decision. In most cases, patients trust their doctor's recommendations. Hence, this trust that he or she is being referred to a competent specialist must not be taken advantage of by the owner doctor's quest for financial gain. There is also the added concern of being liable for a referred-to doctor's treatment when the referring doctor knew or should have known of the referred-to doctor's shortcomings. Always explain to the patient the option of seeing an outside specialist if he or she so desires.

Due to the convenience of being in the same location and the comfort of not having to start a new relationship with a new office, the patient will most likely opt to stay with the practice. Keep in mind that an "overnight success" may take 20 years to achieve. This model is highly adaptable to most practice situations. As always, seek proper professional consultation as needed to properly guide you in such an undertaking.

26

Forms

The forms contained in this chapter are only examples. Do not use them without the advice of your malpractice insurance company and/or local legal counsel to ensure compliance with your state's requirements.

General Release for Dental Treatment (May Be Adapted for Patient by Eliminating the First Sentence)

I, _____ *parent or guardian name* _____, am the _____ *parent/ guardian of patient name* _____. I hereby authorize the doctor to perform any and all forms of dental treatment, medication, and therapy (with my prior consent) that may be indicated in connection with [*name of patient*] and further authorize and consent that the doctor choose and employ such assistance as he or she deems fit. I also understand that dental treatment and the use of anesthetic agents embodies a certain risk. If I have any questions or concerns, I will ask.

Signature_____ Date_____

Relationship_____

Witness_____ Date_____

Professional Responsibility in Dentistry: A Practical Guide to Law and Ethics, Second Edition. Joseph P. Graskemper.
© 2023 John Wiley & Sons, Inc. Published 2023 by John Wiley & Sons, Inc.

Consent for Pulpal Debridement and Endodontic Treatment (Root Canal Tooth #_____)

The purpose of endodontic (root canal) treatment is an attempt to save a tooth rather than to remove it. Although treatment has a high degree of success, it cannot be guaranteed. Pulpal debridement is the removal of the nerve within the tooth and the placement of medication to relieve pain. Sometimes the tooth may need to be reopened and remedicated. Occasionally, the tooth that had root canal treatment may require retreatment, surgery, or even extraction. Endodontic treatment is usually a nonsurgical procedure, but there are inherent risks and limitations such as, but not limited to, file separation (breakage), perforation of the root, calcification of canals, underfilling and overfilling of the canals, and the loss of the tooth. In addition, the porcelain on crowns (caps) can break upon making entry to the root canals. This may necessitate replacement of the crown.

In some cases, a surgical approach is necessary. There may be other complications such as, but not limited to, pain, bleeding, swelling, or infection. In addition, other complications such as sinus involvement, gum recession, numbness or tingling of the lips, face, tongue, or gums are possible. Before any treatment is undertaken, the reason for surgical treatment will be fully explained, including alternative modes of treatment.

Consent is hereby given for the use of local anesthetics, sedation, analgesia, and the use of any materials necessary to fill the root canal as deemed appropriate by the judgment of the dentist. Consent is also given to perform any necessary endodontic procedure that has been fully explained to me. The endodontic (root canal) procedure has been explained to me and I am satisfied that I understand what is to be done. Alternative treatments, including nontreatment, have been explained to me. Costs for the root canal have been explained. I have been given an opportunity to ask questions, and any questions have been answered to my satisfaction. After treatment, the tooth should be restored as soon as possible, usually with a crown (cap). A separate fee will be charged for the restoration.

Signature_____ Date_____

Witness_____ Date_____

Consent for Oral Surgery (Extraction of Tooth # _____)

The oral surgery procedure (extraction) to be performed has been explained to me as well as the alternatives and the ramifications of not having the tooth extracted. I consent to the oral surgery indicated and to other surgery deemed necessary or advisable by the judgment of the dentist, at the time of surgery, in conjunction with the planned surgery. I also consent to the use of local anesthetics, sedation, and analgesia as deemed necessary by the judgment of the dentist during the planned procedure.

I understand that occasionally there are complications associated with surgery. The more common complications are, but are not limited to, pain, infection, swelling, bleeding, bruising, and discoloration; temporary or permanent numbness, pain, burning, or tingling of the lip, check, tongue, chin, gums, and/or teeth; bone fracture; sinus involvement; temporal mandibular joint (TMJ) involvement; delayed healing; change in the bite; that the root fragment may fracture and possibly be left in the jaw; and that there may be damage to adjacent teeth and/or restorations.

I understand there is no warranty or guarantee as to any result and/or cure. Alternative treatments, including nontreatment, have been explained to me. Approximate costs for the surgery have been explained. I have been given an opportunity to ask questions, and any questions have been answered to my satisfaction. I have been informed of the postsurgical care I will need to provide.

Signature_____ Date_____

Witness_____ Date_____

Consent for Periodontal Surgery (Gum Surgery at Tooth # or Area_____)

The periodontal (gum) surgery procedure to be performed has been explained to me, as well as alternatives, including nontreatment. I consent to the periodontal surgery indicated and other surgery deemed necessary or advisable by the judgment of the dentist during the planned procedure. I also consent to the use of local anesthetics, sedation, and analgesia as deemed necessary by the judgment of the dentist during the planned procedure.

I understand that occasionally there are complications associated with periodontal surgery. The more common complications are, but are not limited to, swelling, bleeding, numbness, pain, burning or tingling of the lip, check, tongue, chin, gums, and/or teeth; recession of the gum tissue (the teeth may look longer); hot, cold, sweet sensitivity (although this may decrease with time); exposure of crown margins (which may necessitate replacing the crowns); and tooth mobility, drifting, or loss. I understand that the periodontal surgery cannot guarantee I will keep my teeth or have them for my entire life.

I have been informed that I will need regular maintenance visits (on average, every three months) to help maintain my gums; however, it also is not a guarantee. Alternative treatments, including nontreatment, have been explained to me. The approximate cost for the periodontal surgery has been explained. I also understand the need for proper home care to help in maintaining my teeth. I have been given an opportunity to ask, question, and any questions have been answered to my satisfaction. I have been informed of the postsurgical care I will need to provide.

Signature_____ Date_____

Witness_____ Date_____

General Consent for Surgical and Invasive Procedures

I, _____ *patient name* _____, authorize and consent Dr. _____ *Dr's name* _____ to provide the following treatment: _____ *name of treatment*

_____

_____

I have been made aware of the following risks, but not limited to: _____

_____

_____

_____

I have been made aware of the following alternatives, including nontreatment: _____

_____

_____

_____

I consent to the use of local anesthetics, sedation, and analgesia as deemed necessary by the judgment of the dentist during the planned procedure. I understand there is no warranty or guarantee as to the result and/or cure. The approximate costs for the procedure/treatment have been explained. I have been given an opportunity to ask questions, and any questions have been answered to my satisfaction. I have been informed of the postsurgical care I will need to provide.

Signature_____ Date_____

Witness_____ Date_____

Refusal of Treatment / Referral

I hereby refuse treatment or referral to a specialist for the treatment of_____ _____

_____ _____.

I understand the need for the treatment or referral, and by refusing I accept all responsibility for any consequences of my decision, including loss of the tooth/teeth and other illnesses. The risks of my decision have been explained to me, and any questions have been answered to my satisfaction.

Signature_____ Date_____

Witness_____ Date_____

Termination Letter (Send by Certified Mail, Return Receipt Requested)

Date _____

Dear _____,

I will no longer be able to treat you as my patient effective _____ *date* _____.
Our doctor–patient relationship will be terminated as of _____ *date* _____
because _____*insert a nonantagonistic statement that will not inflame the patient (loss or breakdown of trust, failure to fulfill financial obligations, numerous missed appointments affecting care, etc.).* _____

I must inform you that although you are in a stable condition, you are still in need of dental care. I will be available for emergency care only for the next _____*amount of time (2–4 weeks)* _____.

You may contact _____ *insert name of local dental society* _____ for a new dentist of your choice. With a written notification, I will release and forward copies of your dental records to your new dentist. This will be provided to you at no charge.

The balance that you owe for dental services that have been provided is: _____*insert what you think is a reasonable amount and how you expect it to be paid, including writing off the balance* _____.

Sincerely,

_____

What You Should Know about Financing Your Dental Treatment

FEDERAL TRUTH IN LENDING DISCLOSURE STATEMENT FOR PROFESSIONAL
SERVICES RENDERED

RE: John Smith

Dear Mr. Smith:

In order to comply with the "Truth in Lending Act" and the requirements of Regulation Z, we are required by law to retain a signed copy of this payment schedule in your files, even though no interest or carry charge is included in the following amounts:

Professional Fee for John's Treatment: $500.00
Of which I am responsible for the following: $500.00
Less Initial Fee = $200.00
Financed Amount = $300.00

It is agreed that the **Financed Amount** will be paid in **3** consecutive installments of **$100.00** each, due on the **15th** day of each month beginning 12-15-23 and continue until the **Financed Amount** is paid in full with a final payment of **$100.00.**

This Contract Is to be Paid In Full by 2-15-24

Payer also has the option of paying off the **Balance** before the time stated. Payer also understands that additional treatment may be needed at the time treatment is rendered such that the **Amount Financed** may change accordingly, with payer's consent.

In the event the **Amount Financed** is not paid in a timely manner, all amounts become due and payable and a monthly service charge of 1.5% or a minimum of $1.00 will be charged. Any costs of collection will be added to the balance due. It has been explained to me and I understand that I am responsible for the entire **Professional Fee,** including any unpaid insurance balance.

Signature of Parent or Person

Financially Responsible _____ Date_____

Print Name _____

Authorization for Release of Dental Records

I, _____ *name of patient or guardian* _____, hereby authorize and request
_____*insert name and address of doctor and/or practice* _____ to release,
disclose, and give copies of any and all x-rays, records, and information concerning *name of
patient* _____ to:

Name _____

Address _____

City, State, Zip Code _____

Phone Number _____

In consideration of such disclosure on the part of the above-named person, I hereby release them
from any and all liability arising from such disclosure.

I hereby consent to have my x-rays and any other necessary or requested records to be sent to
Dr. *__name__* in a regular un-encrypted format. I understand that this is an open un-encrypted
unsecured e-mail network and all risks associated with such e-mail.

Sign_____ Date _____

Signature of Parent or Guardian_____ Date _____

Photography Authorization

I, _____*patient name*_____ hereby consent to having my photograph taken. I understand and agree to have the photograph published, duplicated or sent electronically in an open un-encrypted and unsecured email network, with the acknowledgment that the photo may NOT be recalled due to the media used or the photo published, duplicated or sent for use in a professional article, journal or book. In consideration of such disclosure on the part of the above-named person, I hereby release _____ *name of dentist and practice*_____ from any and all liability arising from such disclosure.

Sign_____   Date _____

Release of All Claims

(consult your insurance company or local attorney before use, each jurisdiction may differ)

GENERAL RELEASE

For valuable consideration, the receipt and sufficiency of which are hereby acknowledged, _____*patient's name*_____ ("Releasor"), who lives at _____*patient's Address*_____, does hereby releases, and forever discharges _____*dentist and practice name*___ ("Releasee"), maintaining an address at _____*practice address*_____, Releasee's agents, servants, successors, heirs, executors, administrators, and personal representatives, of and from all, and all manner of, actions, causes of action, including claims for malpractice or professional misconduct, suits, proceedings, debts, dues, contracts, judgments, damages, claims, and demands whatsoever in law or equity, which Releasor ever had, now has, or which Releasor's heirs, executors, administrators, or personal representatives hereafter can, shall, or may have for or by reason of any matter, cause, or thing whatsoever, from the beginning of time to the date of the execution of this release.

It is further agreed that this release does not constitute an admission of any liability, negligence, malpractice, or wrongdoing on the part of the Releasee or its agents.

It is further agreed that the terms of this release are confidential. During the time and thereafter, _____*patient's name*_____ agrees to take no action (written or oral) which is intended, or would reasonably be expected, to harm _____*dentist's and practice name*_____ its/their reputation or which would reasonably be expected to lead to unwanted or unfavorable publicity to the _____*dentist's and practice name*_____.

IN WITNESS WHEREOF, I have executed this Release this day of

_____

(Signature of Releasor)

_____

(Print Name)

STATE OF NEW YORK:

SS:_____

County of _____

On this _____day of _____, 2022, before me, the undersigned, a notary public in and for the said state, personally appeared_____, personally known to me or proved to me on the basis of satisfactory evidence to be the individual(s) whose name(s) is(are) subscribed to the within instrument and acknowledge to me that he/she/they executed the same in his/her/their capacity(ies), and that by his/her/their signature(s) on the instrument, the individual(s) or the person upon behalf of which the individual(s) acted, executed the instrument.

Anti-defamation Clause

I, _____*patient name*_____agree to take no action (written or oral) which is intended, or would reasonably be expected, to harm __*dentist/dental office*__ its/their/his/her reputation or which would reasonably be expected to lead to unwanted or unfavorable publicity to the _____ *dentist/dental office* _____.

Epidemic/Pandemic Dental Treatment Information Form

I _____ *(patient's name)* _____, knowingly and willingly consent to having dental treatment completed during the _____ *name of pandemic* _____ pandemic. I understand the _____ *name of pandemic* _____ has a long incubation period during which carriers of the virus may not show symptoms and could still be highly contagious. Dental procedures create water spray (aerosols) which is one of the ways disease can spread. The ultra-fine nature of the spray can linger in the air for several minutes to hours, which can transmit the virus. Therefore, with the use of ultrasonic cleaning and handpiece spray, we use an extra-oral, high-volume suction that greatly diminishes the exposure to the aerosols created. We also have installed HEPA quality air filters and an air scrubber for the entire office. I understand I have an elevated risk of contracting the virus simply be being in a public setting. Dental offices, while being meticulously cleaned and disinfected, can still present a risk of virus transmission.

_____ *(Patient's Name)* _____   _____ *(Date)*_____

You can also put in questions concerning the patient's health, travels, and possible past exposures and current testing if available.

Index